CANCER
THE HEALTHY OPTION

Born in Wolverhampton in1943, Terry Moule was educated at Tettenhall
College and attended the British College of Naturopathy and Oesteopathy
where, at the age of 20, he was the youngest ever
graduate. He has spent a number of years practising as a
naturopath and has made his name in the treatment of sports injuries and
helping the individual cope with the crisis of cancer. He has been president
of the British Naturopathic Association, has featured regularly on television
and radio and has written many articles on the subject of health.

Terry has been married for 35 years. He lives in Colwall, Worcestershire and
practices in London, St Albans and Worcestershire.

By the same author

Fit for sport

CANCER
THE HEALTHY OPTION

TERRY MOULE
WITH PAMELA BROOKS

WITH AN INTRODUCTION BY BOB WILSON

KYLE CATHIE LIMITED

First published in Great Britain in 2000 by
Kyle Cathie Limited
122 Arlington Road
London NW1 7HP
general.enquiries@kyle-cathie.com

ISBN 1 85626 357 6

Copyright © 2000 by Terry Moule

Designed and typeset by Geoff Hayes
Edited by Georgina Burns
Production by Lorraine Baird and Sha Huxtable

Terry Moule is hereby identified as the author of this work in accordance with Section 77 of the Copyright, Designs and Patents Act 1988.

A CIP catalogue record for this book is available from the British Library.

Printed and bound in Great Britain by Parliamentary Press, London.

contents

Dedication and acknowledgements

Introduction by Bob Wilson 12

Foreword 14

Cancer is a crisis 14

Making decisions 15

The naturopathic approach 15

Orthodox treatment 17

Changing the mental approach 18

All about health 19

Chapter 1 **Health as normality and the energy equation 20**

Medicine in history 20

Medicine today 21

The body and the immune system 21

Energy 22: *biomagnetic energy 23, resonant energy 23, chemical energy 23, life energy 24, The energy equation 24*

Smoking 26

The energy bank 27: *cheques 27 , credit cards 27, direct debits 28, Balancing the accounts, 28, using credit cards 28, when the energy bank becomes low 29,* overdrafts and bankruptcy 29, *treating the disease 30*

Personal responsibility 31

Chapter 2 **Cancer: its development and symptoms 32**

The development of cancerous cells 32

Signs of cancer 33

Detecting cancer 33: *self-examination 34, scans 34, biopsies 36, metastasis 37, staging 37*

Common types of cancer – facts and figures: *bladder cancer 38, bowel cancer 38, brain cancer 38, breast cancer 39, cervical cancer 39, lung cancer 39, lymphoma cancer 40, prostate cancer 40, skin cancer 40, testicular cancer 41*

Warning signs of the more common types of cancer: *bladder cancer 41, bowel cancer 41, brain cancer 41, breast cancer 42, cervical cancer 42, lung cancer 42, lymphoma cancer 43, prostate cancer 43, skin cancer 43, testicular cancer 43*

Diagnosis of the more common types of cancer: *bladder cancer 44, bowel cancer 44, brain cancer 45, breast cancer 45, cervical cancer 45, lung cancer 46, lymphoma cancer 46, prostate cancer 46, skin cancer 46, testicular cancer 46*

Chapter 3 **The treatment options: orthodox medicine 47**

Time 47

Making a choice 48

Seeing an oncologist 48

Orthodox medicine 49: surgery 49, radiotherapy 51, chemotherapy 54

Orthodox treatment of the more common types of cancer 58:

bladder cancer 58, bowel cancer 60, brain cancer 61, breast cancer 62, cervical cancer 63, lung cancer 64, lymphoma cancer 65, prostate cancer 66, skin cancer 67, testicular cancer 68

Side-effects of orthodox treatment of the more common types of cancer 68: *bladder cancer 68, bowel cancer 69, brain cancer 70, breast cancer 70, cervical cancer 71, lung cancer 72, lymphoma cancer 73, prostate cancer 73, skin cancer 74, testicular cancer 74*

Chapter 4 **The treatment options: alternative and complementary therapies 75**

Alternative and complementary therapies 75:

Alternative therapies *76, Naturopathy 76,*

Complementary therapy: *acupuncture 78, Alexander technique 79, aromatherapy 80, Bach flower remedies 81, colour therapy 81, healing (hands on or off) 82, herbalism 83, homeopathy 84, kinesiology 85, magnetic therapy 86, massage 86, reflexology 87, reiki 88, yoga 88*

The approach of treatment 89

Avoiding side-effects 90

Re-creation of health 91

The ideal approach 92

Chapter 5 **Nutrition 94**

Quality food and the difficulties of obtaining it 94: *minerals 94, changing soil structure 95, water in the plant cycle 98, animal foods 98, artificial fertiliser versus the organic approach 99, why organic is better for you 100, eating in season 100*

Energy and elimination 101

The balance of foodstuffs 101

Starting to re-create health 103: *first two weeks 103, chemotherapy diet 105, general diet 105*

Detoxification 107

Food preparation 107: *raw 108, steaming 108 , grilling 108, stir-frying 108,* microwaving 108, *other methods 109*

The healthy approach to eating 109

Supplementation: *chemical isolates versus food state minerals 109*

Water 112: *tap water 112, bottled water 112, filtered water 113, distilled water 113, reverse osmosis 114, cold vaporisation 114*

Supplementation and the concept of eating to get well 115

Eating for life 117

Recipes 118–150

Chapter 6 Exercise and structure 151

Posture 151

Structure 152

Why we need exercise 153

Sensible exercise 154

Cancer and exercise 154: *starting to exercise 155, increasing the amount you exercise 158, if you're used to exercise 160*

Breathing exercises 163

Sex 164

Chapter 7 Psychological, emotional and spiritual matters 165

Fear 165

Living in the present 168

Using the mind positively 168

Viewing everything for the best 169

Love 170

Starting within ourselves 170

The people around us 171

Destressing techniques 173: *Eeman technique 173, thinking about what you do as you do it 174, other techniques 175*

Spiritual matters 175

Chapter 8 **The whole person and cancer by Peter Wallace 177**

Cancer Help Centre lessons 177

Cancer people are wonderful people 178

We are all connected 178

Choosing for you 179

You are not alone 179

Ask and listen 180

A loving environment 181

Nothing happens by chance 182

World traditions of reflection 182

Ask a friend to help by listening to you 183

Enjoy your choices 184

Postscript 185

Chapter 9 **Managing cancer and the re-creation of health 186**

Increasing your energy income 187: *nutritional 187, structural 187,
emotional 188, decreasing expenditure 188*

Net result 189

The right to choose 189

The only real antidote to disease 190

Glossary of terms 191

Appendix 1 **Where to find alternative & complementary practitioners 195**

Appendix 2 **RDA of vitamins and minerals for healthy adults and for adults with cancer 205**

Appendix 3 **Approximate correlation between food state nutrients and traditional supplements 208**

Appendix 4 **Self-help groups 209**

Appendix 5 **Suppliers 215**

Index 216

I would like to dedicate this book to my father, Tom W. Moule, one of the great pioneers of naturopathy and health creation in this country, as a way of thanking him for his love, education and experience which enabled me to carry on in his giant footsteps.

I would also like to dedicate this book to my great friend Roy Castle whose courage and attitude during his own crisis with cancer was an inspiration to everyone.

Acknowledgements

Firstly I would like to thank Pamela Brooks who was a wonderful help in putting this book together under urgent circumstances. I would like to thank my friend and colleague Peter Wallace for his contributions and also for the help he has given me in my mental and spiritual progress and also thank my friend and colleague Eric Llewellyn for his continuing and important input into my nutritional knowledge and pursuit of health. Last and by no means least I would like to thank Rosalie Dickinson for the wonderful gift of Rapha, in which she played such a great part, and for her present and continuing help with all things related to health creation and well-being of the whole person. Finally, I would like to thank Bob Wilson for his kindness, interest and effort in writing the introduction.

Introduction

When my daughter Anna was diagnosed, at the age of twenty-six, with a very rare form of cancer, life as we had known it suddenly took on new priorities. Yes, it was a crisis, or a *turning point*, so succinctly put within the pages of this book by Terry Moule.

To a certain degree she knew a lot – not all, but was prepared to take on the impostor that is cancer head-on. In her words, it would take her *kicking and screaming*. Even with Anna's insight and courage, there was so much that came as a shock to her and to us, and emotions often included not just raw fear but uncontrollable anger.

For five years Anna's life – our family life – took on the roller-coaster pattern so familiar to many others who have faced a similar problem. The learning curve can be very sharp and how one copes depends almost entirely on the patient and those closest to them. From the moment of diagnoses, Anna wanted answers and searched books and the internet for information. Sometimes it helped; sometimes it hurt.

With Anna, quality of time and quality of life were always her priorities and the need to be treated as normal, not as someone who was facing a life-threatening illness, was paramount. Love, laughter, fun and having regular *special days* out, or in, were always on the top of her list.

Cancer can be a humbling experience, to some totally devastating and to others the *turning point* in their lives, a crisis which makes them realise what is important and what isn't. It changes the priorities of those sensible enough to see the positive things, rather than the negative and the mundane.

Terry Moule's book covers, in the most comprehensive way, cancer in all its forms, warts and all. It is one of the most valuable publications about this most seemingly frightening of illnesses, inviting an understanding of the problem as a whole. It sets out the options available and encourages the action of choice, whatever path is chosen, whether it is orthodox or alternative. It promotes the creation of health at times of preparation for treatment and after treatment, encouraging patients to take out a stake in their own future.

Every cancer is unique in its course and its effect, but what this book does is help prepare, steel and comfort those who need to choose a determined way of coping with whatever is thrown at them.

It's perhaps a strange thing to admit but taking on and fighting cancer face-to-face can, whatever the outcome, prove to be the most positive, even rewarding of experiences.

Bob Wilson
Co-founder of the Willow Foundation, a charity giving special days to seriously ill young adults

Foreword:
Cancer is a crisis

Cancer is a crisis. The dictionary definition of a crisis is a turning point, and my aim in this book is to help people in this crisis turn in the right direction.

This book is aimed at anybody who has cancer, people who know someone who has it, or anyone who is worried about getting it. It explains what cancer is, what kind of treatments are available (both orthodox and alternative/complementary), what kind of side-effects orthodox treatments have, what you can do to help re-create your own health in terms of nutrition, exercise and emotional/spiritual matters and the importance of understanding how you can create and maintain health, irrespective of whether your choice is orthodox, alternative/complementary, or you choose to have no treatment at all. It also explains where you can go for more detailed information about your particular cancer.

The information will also help family members and carers know what to expect from treatment and work out where the patient may need extra support. However, this book is not specifically aimed at supporting family members, friends and carers. It does not lay down a blueprint for curing cancer and it does not claim to cure you – it will help you find the right route for you and give you the facts so that you can make an informed choice. It helps to give you, the individual, the ability to make this choice and empower yourself to give your body every chance of creating and maintaining health.

While the disease is one of the most traumatic things that can happen to anybody, in my thirty-seven years practising as a naturopath I've seen that the way that cancer is managed and the decisions you choose can make a huge difference to the long-term effect the disease has on your quality and term of life.

Making decisions

You can only make decisions when you have all the information, and this book will give you the simple statistical information and facts so you can see the problem as part of the whole picture, then make your decision about the best treatment for you.

If you have already started a course of treatment and are partway – or even fully – down the line of orthodox therapy, this book can still help you. There's a huge amount you can do to help your body deal with the remainder of its treatment, and to rebuild it and restore health after the treatment has finished.

Healing is a combination of ancient and current wisdom. The unique angle of this book is my own experience, particularly over the last two years, during which I have seen an increased number of cancer patients. I can't treat or cure you, but I can help you help yourself to regain and maintain health, particularly by using a nutritional formula. I've had more experience than anyone with this naturopathic approach and it's time to share that knowledge so that you too can take the healthy option.

The naturopathic approach

What I mean by the healthy option is the naturopathic approach – that is, giving the individual a chance to empower him or herself to re-create health by liberating the natural healing energies in the body. This can only be achieved by understanding all the options available regarding treatment, making an educated choice from those options and then using the naturopathic approach to nutrition, controlled exercise and a positive mental attitude to support and maintain the approach you decide upon.

A naturopath is someone whose practice is based on four principles:

• The individuality of the patient

• Trying to establish and treat the cause(s) of the condition, not just the symptoms

• The belief that everyone has the potential within their body to heal themselves – this is often described as *vis medicatrix natuari* or 'the healing forces of nature'

• Treating the whole person and not just the local area of the body that may be affected

Medical treatment will attack the symptoms using various methods that I will describe later in the book, but will not do anything to remove the cause. The naturopathic approach is to increase the energy available in the body, which will enable the immune system to function and thus, by re-creating health, help to remove the cause. Once the cause has been removed, the body will be able to maintain its natural preventative methods on an ongoing basis.

The main difference between the naturopathic and orthodox approach is that with the naturopathic approach you, the individual, are at all times in control of your own future and the maintenance of your own health. Naturopathy gives you the chance to work with nature and take a positive approach to the creation of health. The treatment of a symptom is something that is done *to* you, but the creation of health is something that is done *by* you – and in my years of practice I've seen that nothing is impossible.

Orthodox treatment

We have been reared in a society medically controlled by a health service which is, in fact, disease rather than health-based. Scientific medicine has led us to a point where a condition must be accurately diagnosed so that a very specific treatment can be prescribed. Misdiagnosis can actually cause death since many drugs, if wrongly used, can have fatal side-effects or direct effects. This approach has meant that diagnosis has become the king of the medical approach.

Millions have been spent in developing diagnostic techniques and equipment to enable better and better pinpointing of the specific disease. These techniques and equipment are very accurate, but they have to diagnose an ever-increasing range of diseases. These diseases are frequently the result of the side-effects of chemical treatment while there are many new conditions which cannot actually be treated by existing medicine. There are viruses which are currently untreatable by any known means, leaving the body to deal with the problem by itself – which it can.

It is a shame that there is such a long and arduous road between the point of realising that there is a problem – such as cancer – and the point of understanding that the body can deal with it and heal itself if the underlying causes are looked at.

As a result of diagnostic medicine, we are all very aware of the disease names, the potential treatment for them and, sometimes, their possible causes. This has led us to concentrate on the disease and its symptoms and develop a quest for more and more knowledge about them – which in turn leads to a negative frame of mind, where we look at the problems rather than the causes. This negative frame of mind has a physical effect on the body, and this is particularly true when it comes to cancer.

Changing the mental approach

The naturopathic approach to this – which I believe is the healthy option –
is to change your mental approach entirely, by taking disease completely out
of the equation. Instead of thinking about having treatment for cancer,
think instead of re-creating and maintaining health. Every time you think
about cancer you empower that condition within the body; equally, every
time you think about health, you empower that concept and state of well-
being within the body.

Seeing health, feeling health and being health is so much better than
the opposite; and it becomes easier as you get more used to this concept
and can reap the benefits of using the power of the mind constructively
and positively.

Even if you are having medical treatment for cancer, such as
chemotherapy or surgery, leave the treatment to the medical profession and
concentrate your mind on creating health to support whatever your body
has to deal with. At all costs, avoid taking the treatment into part of your
mental approach.

If you do, what it means is that in the present all you tend to be dragged
into thinking about, talking about and, above all, fearing and worrying
about is the cancer problem itself. The alternative is to concentrate on and
respond to health, in the present, and this means that there is an instant
change in the body's functions and future potential.

Remember that man is body, mind and spirit. The mind is a key to
unlocking the beneficial effects of both sides of the coin. Being positive is
what we are meant to do, and being positive in the present means that the
past has been accepted and left behind and the future is still there waiting to
be created. Applying positivity to this equation is the step to creating health
and well-being in the future.

All about health

Normal health is where the body's natural energy equation is balanced; when there is an obstruction to the natural energy in the body, it leads to disease. This book will explore what health is, what the obstructions are, and how you can work on them and use your body's energy bank so that it can deal with the symptoms itself.

Cancer is a major problem, but if you accept it, you can do something positive yourself and assert control over the situation; concentrate on the creation of normal function and this will help you cope with everything else. Remember, a crisis is defined as a turning point.

Chapter 1
Health as normality and the energy equation

Cancer is reaching epidemic proportions in modern civilisation. At the moment, one in four people are affected by it. The forecast is that within ten years five out of seven people could be affected by carcinogenic problems of one form or another. Cancer is indeed a disease of civilisation.

In order to understand the mechanism behind the onset of cancer – and all other disease processes – it is first of all important to understand health and how the body can and should function effectively.

Medicine in history

For many thousands of years medicine was practised on the Hippocratic basis of 'Let your medicine be your food and your food be your medicine.' Doctors used herbs, diet and water as the means of creating and maintaining health.

The ancient Chinese had a very effective medical system: the doctor was paid while his patient was well, but if the patient fell ill the doctor was not paid until the patient was once again healthy. This process meant that the aims and objects of every practitioner were to encourage and nurture the state of health of the patient and to spend time on creative and preventative medicine. The best prevention of disease was found to be health, and thus a really effective health service was delivered.

Medicine today

If we look at medicine today, we can see that it has been led down a route of specific treatment for specific symptoms and the removal of those symptoms, rather than the creation of health by the removal of the causes of the disease. Rather than a National Health Service, we have created what is essentially a National Disease Service. If the average GP is asked about the creation of health, his or her first question is likely to be, 'What is wrong with you?'

Sir Robert McCarrison, a former President of the Royal College of Physicians and author of The Wheel of Health, said over thirty years ago that he believed, after many years in medicine, he knew most of what there was to know about disease but almost nothing about health. Sadly, this is still true of many practitioners because of the focus on symptom removal.

The body and the immune system

The body is designed to be able to maintain health and fitness; through control from within it can deal with all the various assaults upon its system that the environment can provide. The immune system is designed to cope with the outward attacks and it can also control from within any abnormal activities which may occur.

Everybody has cancer cells within them, but in the state of balanced health the immune system controls them and the individual is neither aware of the presence of these cells nor suffers any effect.

When the immune system is damaged, it doesn't function properly. Our growing obsession with hygiene means that many of us live in a fairly sterile environment with the result that our immune system is rarely used; and when the immune system becomes low, the development of cancer becomes both a possibility and indeed a probability. So the old-fashioned idea of 'eating a peck of dirt' in our lifetime isn't a bad thing.

When the function of our immune system is lowered due to a drop in energy levels, we get early warning signals such as becoming tired, having headaches and being affected by germs and viruses. Rather than let our bodies deal with them, we try to suppress these warning signs by taking stimulants to combat tirednes, painkillers to relieve headaches and antibiotics to eliminate germs and viruses – the overuse of antibiotics causing the rise of superbugs is well documented, and stimulants and other medication can cause the build-up of toxic waste in the body. A cold should be seen as a safety valve; if we try to suppress it with drugs, it can create other problems (and will also last longer when we stop taking the drugs). We should feel better after a cold but now we have to 'get over it' for some days. What you need to do is to let the body deal with it by reducing your intake of suppressive foods, such as dairy produce in particular, refined carbohydrates and heavily processed foods. Instead, concentrate on organic fruit and salads for a few days to release energy from the digestive and assimilation process, to increase eliminative and immune function. This will remove the cause and therefore the symptoms, and instead of feeling bad you end up feeling better.

Energy

In order to understand the maintenance of health we need to look at energy, which is the key to body function: how it is made available and what happens to it once it is present in the body. The energy cycle and its maintenance are the keystone to continued good health; conversely, the lack of and reduction in available energy is the starting point of the disease process.

Energy, despite many people's perceptions, does not come from food alone. If this were the case, the more food we ate the more energetic we would become. Food is only one part of energy: namely, chemical energy. Life energy is also made up of biomagnetic energy and resonant energy.

Biomagnetic energy

All living objects have a life energy, which is of an electromagnetic nature and which is present as part of the energy of the earth itself; the whole world is magnetically balanced through the poles, although cars, planes, electricity pylons and many other human activities disturb the earth's magnetism.

Biomagnetic energy helps to encourage balanced cell function and works as a shield to external attack. The use of magnets in healing is increasing, and it improves the balance of the body's magnetic field. This helps the body to lower inflammation and improve circulation, and aids the body's overall management system by enabling the body's energy lines to function normally.

Resonant energy

This is the vibrational energy of all living things. In a balanced body, the cells will resonate in harmony and then create life energy. Cell resonance and its balance is very much part of a homeopathic approach to health creation and maintenance. Keeping this harmonic balance at all times is a very important part of the body's total energy picture. Without this, the chemical and other energies (such as nutrition) cannot be fully used within the body's maintenance system.

Chemical energy

Chemical energy – that is, nutrition – is needed to maintain the body in its correct functioning form, so it can carry out the tasks which are required by the muscles, organs and brain to keep the whole structure functioning effectively on a minute-to-minute basis. Chemical energy is particularly important for the immune system as without adequate energy from this source, the human being is not able to tap into the life energy as effectively as he or she needs to in order to maintain health.

Life energy

Life energy – that is, a combination of biomagnetic energy, resonant energy and chemical energy – is like a radio wave. It is available to everyone but, just as with radio receivers, what you hear from the radio wave depends upon the radio receiver itself. The old portable set with its single speaker and low battery lets us know that the music is pleasant – but only just! – while the presenter's voice may be indistinguishable. Conversely the modern stereo set with its good aerial, high quality speakers and surround sound not only interprets the music but every instrument involved in producing the music while the presenter's voice is clearly distinguishable.

Just as the receiver is the critical factor in being able to use the radio wave, your body, acting as a receiver, is critical in your ability to use life energy.

The energy equation

One way of looking at it is to see it as an energy equation: that is, ENERGY equals LIFE ENERGY minus OBSTRUCTIONS. The energy is then paid into the energy bank account (see diagram below).

We have already seen that life energy is made up of biomagnetic, resonant and chemical energy. Similarly, the obstructions can be broken down into three main components: dietetic and nutritional; structural and breathing; and mental, emotional and spiritual. These obstructions and how to deal with them will be covered in later chapters. There are environmental

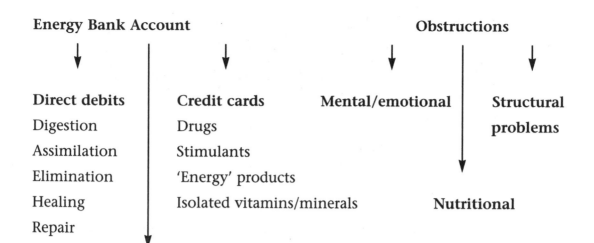

Energy Bank Account　　　　　　　　　　**Obstructions**

Direct debits　　　**Credit cards**　　**Mental/emotional**　　**Structural**
Digestion　　　　　　Drugs　　　　　　　　　　　　　　　　　**problems**
Assimilation　　　　　Stimulants
Elimination　　　　　'Energy' products
Healing　　　　　　　Isolated vitamins/minerals　　　**Nutritional**
Repair

Cheques
40% immediate increase when eyes are open
plus all conscious activities

obstructions as well; these are mainly to do with magnetic disturbances of the earth, such as the area around pylons – which are related to some forms of cancer (such as brain cancer and leukaemia), and pollution, where toxic matter in rainwater affects the food chain. Rain comes down to earth, waters the ground and enters the water table, carrying pollution from the air and absorbing further pollution in the ground. This water is then used by humans and animals alike.

What the energy equation shows is that the amount of energy we have available to use is dependent upon not obstructing our access to the life energy itself.

In order to maintain health it is essential to have a well-controlled diet and nutrition, good posture and body usage with good breathing techniques, and a positive and constructive approach to life, living in the present.

Any imbalance or inadequacy in any of the three obstructional areas will result in a reduced amount of energy available in the body's energy bank. When you consider the sort of nutritional lifestyle that most people follow – fast and refined foods, lots of saturated fats and sugar, and *eating on the hoof* – and the fact that most people don't exercise regularly or have a good knowledge of breathing techniques, and then add in the negativity and stress present in most parts of life and many people's inability to be aware of the present, it's easy to see why the available energy is not adequate to maintain optimum health.

The obstructions are all inter-related. For example, if you stand badly, you compress the thorax, which affects heart and lung functions. This in turn affects the diaphragm, which then affects the colon and the elimination system – which is linked to nutrition and dietetics. When you don't eat or process food properly, you become tense, which often leads to increased stress. Stress causes physical tension, which affects the muscle tone, which then affects your posture and can lead to interference with nerve root function. You therefore stand badly, and the vicious circle starts again.

Stress can work both ways: if you're tense physically, you're likely to be tense mentally as well. And so the obstructions increase.

Smoking

One thing I should mention here is smoking. It's been proven beyond doubt that smoking is a major factor in cancer and general health. It causes lung problems and has an adverse effect on the energy bank. It stops the proper oxygenation of the blood and slows down the body's processes, while the body also has to dissipate the heat of the smoke and get rid of the toxins. Even if you don't smoke personally, passive smoking – where you inhale smoke from other people's cigarettes – can cause cancer. One example of this is Roy Castle, one of the nicest people I've ever met; he never smoked but in his early career he played a lot of clubs and, as a trumpet player, inhaled a great deal of smoke. And he died from lung cancer.

The energy bank

To understand how energy is used, we can consider the analogy of the energy bank, which illustrates where energy goes and how it can be controlled.

ENERGY BANK

CHEQUES/CREDIT CARDS	DIRECT DEBITS
(conscious activity out)	(unconscious activity out)
All conscious activity from the	Assimilation, elimination,
point of awakening	healing and repair

Cheques

The moment we wake up and open our eyes, we increase our energy consumption by 40 per cent. When we're asleep, although the brain is still working it's at an unconscious level. When we open our eyes, we take in outside signals and this conscious activity steps up the amount of work our brain has to do. From this point on, *cheques* are paid out of the energy bank in exchange for all mental and physical activities we undertake. The bigger the activity, the bigger the cheque that comes out of our 'energy bank account'.

Credit cards

We can also use *credit cards* – that is, an artificial means where we borrow money (or energy) to stimulate function (such as by using alcohol and energy drinks) so that we can pay out money (or energy) instantly. This form of credit has to be paid back and is one of the causes of problems in energy usage in the body, as we shall see below.

Direct debits

Direct debits are paid as and when required; they are the unconscious activities which go on to maintain the body in its normal state. That is, the digestion of food which is eaten, its chemical assimilation into the system and, most importantly, the elimination of the waste matters produced after the required nutrients have been taken. The healing and repair processes which involve the immune system function are also paid by direct debit and these again are completely unconscious.

Balancing the accounts

In the ideal state where the obstructions do not interfere with the body's access to energy, there is a high level of income into the energy bank, so all cheque payments can be met and all direct debits paid on demand. Because you will not need a *loan* of energy, you will not need to use *credit cards*.

Sadly, in almost everybody's case there is not adequate money in the bank account because of the obstructions to the energy access.

What happens then? As we have seen before, when energy is low, the body has mechanisms to advise us that something is wrong. Tiredness is one of the first symptoms and we should take it as a hint to stop spending cheques and allow the bank balance to rebuild. If we don't, there will be signs of direct debits not being paid, such as headaches, digestive disorders and a general feeling of malaise.

Using credit cards

If we reduce cheque expenditure and make corrections to our lifestyle to increase the income as soon as we notice these warning signs, the body will soon return to normal function where the cheques and direct debits can be paid. Generally, this does not happen and we resort to credit cards – using stimulants such as coffee, tea, soft drinks, energy drinks and alcohol to artificially stimulate our bodies to allow the cheques to go on being paid.

While this credit card approach of 'pay now, repay later' enables the individual to carry on an unnatural lifestyle, the reduction in the amount of money in the bank means that direct debits cannot be met in full.

When the energy bank becomes low

When direct debits cannot be met in full, it causes three main changes:

• Assimilation of energy (digestion) decreases, which affects the body's ability to use food

• Elimination is reduced, which increases toxicity within the body

• The healing and repair system – particularly the immune system – is reduced in efficiency so it cannot deal, as well, with germs and cell abnormalities

The outcome of these changes is that the body faces increased obstructions to accessing energy and the payment into the bank account is reduced. However, we still keep on spending cheques. As the energy is reduced and the body becomes more toxic and less efficient, further signs of disease and discomfort appear and these are generally controlled by taking chemical substances which prevent us knowing that they are present – and we still keep paying cheques.

Overdrafts and bankruptcy

Eventually the overdraft in the energy bank increases so much that near-bankruptcy is reached and the body's health-maintenance system breaks down. At this point the immune system ceases to function effectively; the body's defence system against germs and cell abnormality is therefore breached, and the onset of serious disease becomes inevitable. Cancer in particular is very much a disease of deficient immune function.

Treating the disease

Once the body has sunk to a *disease* level of function, various forms of treatment are applied. The only way to remove the basic cause of all disease is to rebuild the bank account and control the payment of cheques, to enable the direct debits to be paid and the eliminative system to begin to function again. Only in this way can the body regain its ability to manage its own health and put normal function in place of disease symptoms.

In the case of cancer, chemotherapy, radiotherapy and surgery are the main forms of orthodox treatment; their purpose is to kill or remove the cancerous cells and to prevent their spread to other parts of the body. As scientific and technical knowledge has improved over the years, these forms of treatment have become far more controlled and less punishing in their effect on the body; but unfortunately this approach does nothing to remove the cause of the problem, only the symptom.

In later chapters, we will look at the obstructions to normal function, the types of treatment available and the alternatives to disease treatment.

Personal responsibility

Health is a personal responsibility and nobody can treat or cure another individual. Symptoms can be removed by external treatment but the real cure – health – can only be achieved by a personal awareness of how the body functions, what its needs are and then a dedication of effort to remove the obstructions to normal function to fill up the account in the energy bank and have the ability to pay cheques and direct debits as necessary.

The good news is that the process of disease can be reversed. If you consciously change the obstructions, your body will go back to normal function. Your mental and emotional state is the key to starting this process of reversal. At ground level, you need to control your nutrition to put basic energy into your account. This will help to lift the mental side – and then you can start to make the right decisions about your own treatment.

Chapter 2
Cancer: its development and symptoms

The development of cancerous cells

Our body is made up of millions of cells. Each cell has its own function and they all act in a specific way; a bone cell won't suddenly become a muscle cell and a liver cell won't suddenly become a heart cell.

However, sometimes the normal regulatory mechanism of a cell no longer happens. Normal cells grow to their desired size and space out evenly, only dividing to replace old cells or those that are worn out; they stick together in the right place and self-destruct if they are damaged. A cancerous cell, however has mutated so it will grow as fast as it can and keep multiplying and dividing until a lump or tumour develops; they don't stick together and they don't obey signals from neighbouring cells. By the time the tumour is big enough to be felt, it may contain billions of cells.

The tumour grows until it invades its neighbouring structures, forcing itself through normal tissues and blocking small blood vessels; the normal tissues, once deprived of blood and oxygen in this way, will begin to die off and let the tumour push itself through.

Because cancerous cells don't stick together as normal cells do, they can also break off and spread to another part of the body through the blood stream or lymphatic system, forming secondary cancers. This process is known as metastasis.

This can happen to any type of cell – bone, blood, skin, etc – so there are actually more than 200 different types of cancer. Having said that, half of new cancer cases are accounted for by lung, breast, bowel and prostate forms, and over 65 per cent of all new cancers in the UK are diagnosed to people over the age of 65.

The different types of cancer have different symptoms and respond differently to different treatments.

Signs of cancer

Experts have drawn up a list of signs which can indicate cancer. If you have any of these symptoms, talk to your GP:

- A change in bowel or bladder habits
- A sore that will not heal
- Unusual bleeding or discharge
- Thickening or a lump in a breast (or elsewhere)
- Difficulty in swallowing or indigestion
- An obvious change in a wart or mole
- A nagging cough or hoarseness

However, it is worth remembering that these signs are also often symptoms of other medical problems that are not as serious as cancer – for example, pain on urination may be due to cystitis or a bladder stone. While it is sensible to have yourself checked out, do not develop a fear of cancer. Fear is a major factor in causing bodily imbalance.

Detecting cancer

Certain types of cancer – such as breast, bowel, cervical, ovarian and prostate – may run in families or be more common in later life. You may be offered screening if you have a higher risk of cancer due to your family history or your age. It is important to remember that inherent tendencies can develop unless a positive lifestyle is followed.

Self-examination

Self-examination can help early detection of certain types of cancer:

Breast cancer: lie down with a pillow under your left shoulder and raise your left hand above your head. With the flat part of the fingers of your right hand, carefully examine your left breast. In a circular pattern, start from the outer top, pressing firmly enough to feel the tissue beneath. After one full circle, move an inch and circle again, continuing until you reach the nipple. Check the area above your breast, especially the armpit area, for lumps or hard knots. Squeeze your nipple to check for discharge. Repeat with the right breast.

Testicular cancer: examination is best done after a warm bath or shower, when the scrotal skin relaxes. Support the scrotum in the palm of your hand and examine each testicle by rolling it between your fingers and thumb. Press gently to feel for lumps, swellings, or changes in firmness.

Scans

There are several different types of scans which doctors can use to see tumours. These include:

Barium enema – this is where you are given an enema (through a tube in your back passage which goes into your bowel) containing barium sulphate, a special metallic liquid that shows white on x-rays. The doctor will then take x-ray pictures to see if there are any blockages or lumps. You will not need any anaesthetic but it may give you constipation, so you'll need to drink plenty, and eat more fibre to get rid of the chemicals. This technique is often used for bowel cancer.

CT or cat scan (computerised tomography or computed axial tomography) – this is a special type of scan which takes a cross-sectional picture of part of your body, using a combination of x-rays and a computer. It shows a clearer picture than x-rays alone and minimises the amount of radiation exposure. You lie on a couch which slides backwards and forwards through the scanner (which looks a bit like a large doughnut); it doesn't hurt but you need to lie still and the scanning procedure can take around half an hour, so you may feel a bit stiff afterwards. You can ask for the scan to be stopped at any time, for example if you need to go to the loo or you're about to sneeze. This technique is often used for bowel cancer and brain cancer; it's also good for scanning organs.

MRI (Magnetic Resonance Image) – this is where a powerful magnetic field is used to create a picture of your body. You lie on a couch which slides backwards and forwards through the scanner, which is like a large tube. It's noisy so you may be given ear plugs. As with the CT scan, it doesn't hurt but you need to lie still and the scanning procedure can take between half an hour and an hour, so you may feel a bit stiff afterwards. The technique can be used on any part of the body but is often used for brain cancer and muscle cancer (sarcoma).

X-rays – this is where low doses of electromagnetic energy with short wavelengths are passed through your body to create an image of your bones, organs and internal tissues on a screen or film. You will not need an anaesthetic. This technique is often used for brain cancer, lung cancer and lymphoma.

Angiogram or arteriogram – this is where a special dye is injected into your artery and flows into the blood vessels, showing the position of the tumour when you are x-rayed. It is often used for brain cancer.

Lymphangiogram – this is similar to an angiogram but the special dye is used to outline your lymph nodes. It is used for lymphoma.

Ultrasound – this is a special type of scan where inaudible, ultra-high frequency sound waves can show a picture of your internal organs and the location and size of any tumour. A special jelly will be placed on your skin to help transmit the sound waves and then the scanner is passed over your skin, passing sound waves into your body which bounce back and project the image of your internal organs onto a screen. It doesn't hurt and takes around half an hour. It is often used for breast cancer, prostate cancer and testicular cancer.

Biopsies

Doctors can also take a sample of the tumour – known as a biopsy – and can look at it under a microscope to check whether the cells are cancerous. The sample is usually taken using a fine needle, an endoscope or simply cutting away a small piece of skin or muscle and is a minor procedure. You may be given either a local or a general anaesthetic, depending on the site of the tumour.

Metastasis

Although cancer may form in one particular organ, it may spread from the original site to other parts of the body. This happens when cancer cells break off from the tumour and travel through the blood vessels or lymphatic fluids to another part of the body. Although your immune system may kill these travelling cells, some of the cells may survive and settle, then continue to grow in their new environment. Through the blood vessels, the cancer cells can reach nearly all the tissues in the body. Cancer cells often settle in bones (a process known as bone metastatis) and cause pain; around half of people with cancer (except skin cancer) will suffer from bone metastatis. The most common area affected is the spine, followed by the pelvis, hip, upper leg bones and skull.

Even when secondary cancers form in this way – known as metastasis – they are still called after the part of the body where they originally formed. For example, if breast cancer spreads to the lungs, it is still called breast cancer.

Treatment of the secondary cancers depends on where the primary cancer started, where it has spread to and whether any bones are weakened or broken. Orthodox treatments – which are discussed in greater detail in Chapter 3 – include chemotherapy, radiotherapy and surgery.

Staging

Staging is a way of giving doctors a common language to describe cancers and compare treatment results. One of the most common is the *TNM* system, which stands for *Tumour, Node, Metastatis.*

T describes the size of the primary cancer on a scale of 1-4, with 1 being small and 4 being large. N describes whether the lymph nodes have any cancer cells on a scale of 0-3, with 0 meaning that no lymph nodes have cancer cells and 3 meaning that many lymph nodes have cancer cells. M describes whether the cancer has spread elsewhere (metastasis), with 0 meaning that it hasn't and 1 meaning that it has.

Common types of cancer – the facts and figures

Bladder cancer
- The fifth most common cancer in the UK
- The fifth most common cancer in men
- Affects three times as many men as women worldwide
- More than half of cases occur in the over-70s
- Risk is increased by smoking or bladder infections by a parasitic worm called *Schistosoma haematobium* (mainly found in parts of Africa and the Middle East).

Bowel cancer
- Cancer of the large bowel (colon and rectum) is the second most common cancer in the UK
- Rare in the under-40s and more common in the elderly
- The risk is increased by a low-fibre, high-fat diet; being overweight; and drinking lots of alcohol
- Most cases are not diagnosed until it has spread beyond the bowel
- Only 40 per cent of patients survive. It is important to concentrate on being one of these 40 per cent

Brain cancer
- 4000 new cases in the UK each year
- Most common in under-10s and those aged 50-60

• Eleventh most common cancer in men and fifteenth most common cancer in women in the UK

Breast cancer

• Most common cancer in UK women – accounts for 25 per cent of all female cancers

• The risk increases with age – it's rare in under-35s and 80 per cent of breast cancers occur in post-menopausal women

• Men can get it too; there are 200 cases a year in the UK

• With tumours less than 2cm in size, your survival rate for 5 years is likely to be 90 per cent; a tumour larger than 5cm in size has a 5-year survival rate of around 60 per cent

• Risk factors may include long-term use of the contraceptive pill, high alcohol intake and a high-fat diet; 5-10 per cent of cases may be genetic

• Approximately 14,000 women a year die in the UK from breast cancer, although the figure is falling

Cervical cancer

• Second most common cancer in women worldwide

• Eighth most common cancer in UK women

• The risk is related to sexual activity starting before age 18 or having a large number of sexual partners, plus smoking

Lung cancer

• The most common cancer in the world

• The risk increases with age – it's uncommon in under-40s

• 90 per cent of cases are caused by smoking; other risk factors include industrial exposure to carcinogens such as asbestos

• There are two types: non-small cell lung cancer (NSCLC – accounts for 80 per cent of cases) and small cell lung cancer (SCLC – accounts for 20 per cent of cases). The difference between them is based on the behaviour of the cells

Lymphoma cancer

• Develops in the lymphatic system (the part of the body's immune system that fights diseases and infection)

• Non-Hodgkin's lymphoma is the seventh most common cancer in the UK

Prostate cancer

• Second most common form of fatal cancer in men – over 10,000 men in the UK die each year from it

• More likely to affect the over-60s

• Can grow for up to 10 years before detection

• Affects 1 in 12 men

• 70–80 per cent of patients with early cancer survive for more than ten years after treatment

• The risk is increased by a diet high in animal fat and low in vitamin A; sexually acquired infections (particularly at a young age); and exposure to heavy metals (particularly cadmium)

Skin cancer

• Most common cancer in many parts of the world

• Three types: basal cell, squamous cell and melanoma

• Among 20-34-year-olds, it is the third most common cancer in women and fourth most common cancer in men

• The risk is linked to high sun exposure

- Those most at risk have fair or red hair, pale skin, freckles and burn easily
- White people are 40 times more likely to have it than coloured people
- If detected early, it has a 99 per cent cure rate

Testicular cancer
- The most common cancer in the UK in men aged between 20 and 35
- 96 per cent of cases can be cured if caught at an early stage; 80 per cent of tumours that have spread can be cured; and 60 per cent of large-volume tumours can be cured – remember to be one of the 60 per cent
- Boys born with an undescended testicle have a greater risk

Warning signs of the more common types of cancer

Bladder cancer
- Blood in the urine – may disappear for days or weeks but will come back; is not usually painful
- Difficulty in passing urine
- Painful spasms in the bladder

Bowel cancer
- Persistent change in bowel habit (diarrhoea or constipation)
- Blood in the stool (either bright red or black)
- Persistent stomach discomfort
- Loss of weight for unknown reason
- A lump in the abdomen

Brain cancer
- Headaches that are worse in the morning and ease during the day

- Fits
- Weakness, loss of feeling in the arms or legs, difficulty walking
- Drowsiness
- Abnormal changes in vision
- Changes in personality, memory or speech

Breast cancer
- Changes in the shape, appearance and feel of your breasts
- Lump in one breast or armpit which is new or different from the other side
- Puckering or dimpling in the skin
- Discomfort or pain in one breast that differs from normal
- Nipple discharge, rash or a change in nipple position

Cervical cancer
- Symptoms are associated with more advanced stages of cancer – not the early stages or pre-cancerous changes (which will be picked up through the smear test)
- Abnormal bleeding – between regular menstrual periods or after sexual intercourse
- Increased vaginal discharge

Lung cancer
- Shortness of breath
- Persistent pain in the chest
- Persistent cough or coughing up blood
- Loss of appetite, weight loss and general tiredness

Lymphoma cancer

• Painless swelling in the lymph nodes – underarm, neck and groin
• Fever, tiredness
• Night sweats
• Itching

Prostate cancer

• Difficulty or pain in urinating
• Urinating more frequently
• Blood in your urine (rare)
• Pain in your back or hips

Skin cancer

• Growth or change in moles
• Ragged outline of mole
• Different colours within a mole
• Moles with reddish edges or inflammation
• Moles that bleed, ooze or crust

Testicular cancer

• A lump in either testicle
• Enlargement in the testicle
• A feeling of heaviness or sudden collection of fluid in the scrotum
• A dull ache in the groin or abdomen

Diagnosis of the more common types of cancer

Bladder cancer

Your GP will ask for a urine sample and will conduct an internal examination – the rectum in men and the vagina in women. He or she may then refer you to a bladder specialist called an urologist, who may ask you to have further tests. These may include:

• Blood test – this is to check your overall health, whether you have anaemia and how well your kidneys are functioning
• Chest x-ray – this is to check that your heart and lungs are healthy
• Intravenous urogram – this is an x-ray which shows up any abnormalities in the kidneys, bladder and urinary system
• Cystoscopy – this is where the doctor looks directly into your bladder using a thin tube with a light on the end (called a cystoscope), examines the lining of the bladder and removes a sample of tissues which are then checked for cancer cells

Bowel cancer

Your GP will give you a full physical examination and blood tests. Other tests you may be given include:
• Endoscopy – this is where the doctor looks into your colon through a special tube (an endoscope) to check for suspicious signs
• Barium enema – you will be given an enema containing barium, a special liquid that shows white on x-rays, and then x-ray pictures will be taken of your bowel to show if there are any blockages or lumps
• CT (computerised tomography) – scan of your abdomen – which shows you in cross-section – to check if the tumour has spread

Brain cancer

Your GP will refer you to a specialist, who will do a neurological examination to check your alertness, muscle strength, co-ordination, reflexes and response to pain. The specialist will also check your eyes in case a tumour causes swelling by pressing on the nerve connecting your eye and your brain. Depending on the results of the tests, he may ask for others, including:

• CT (computerised tomography) scan of your brain (in cross-section)

• MRI (Magnetic Resonance Image) scan of your brain

• Skull x-ray – this may show changes in the bones caused by a tumour

• Angiogram or arteriogram – a special dye is injected into an artery and flows into the blood vessels in the brain, showing the position of the tumour on x-ray

Breast cancer

A mammogram – a special x-ray that can detect very small lumps in the breast – may show if there is a tumour. In the UK, mammograms are routinely offered to the over-50s. You may then have an ultrasound scan, a biopsy (where a sample of the lump is removed and investigated in a laboratory) or needle aspiration (where fluid containing cells from an area of the lump is removed through a fine needle and investigated in a laboratory) to check for cancerous cells.

Cervical cancer

Women aged 20–64 in the UK have a regular screening test called a smear test. A wooden spatula scrapes cells from the cervix which are then analysed in a laboratory. If any cells are abnormal, you will have a repeat smear. If there are still concerns, your doctor will use a special microscope called a colposcope to look at your cervix and may remove a small amount of tissues (biopsy).

Lung cancer

You may be given a chest x-ray. This is usually followed by a bronchoscopy or mediastinascopy, where a thin flexible tube is put down your airways and a sample of suspicious tissue (biopsy) is taken.

Lymphoma cancer

Your doctor may give you blood tests and x-rays of the chest, bones, liver and spleen. If a lymph node is enlarged, the doctor may remove it under anaesthetic (biopsy) to check the cells. If it's cancerous, the doctor needs to know how far it has spread and will give you a lymphangiogram – an x-ray using a special dye to outline the lymph nodes and vessels.

Prostate cancer

Your doctor will give you a rectal examination to assess your prostate – located below the bladder. If it feels abnormal he will send you to a specialist who will give you an ultrasound to detect any abnormality and measure its size. The specialist may also take a biopsy (tissue sample) using a thin needle. There is a screening blood test which measures the level of a substance in the blood called prostate specific antigen (PSA) but the test is not very accurate.

Skin cancer

The doctor will remove part or all of the suspicious-looking growth (biopsy) and check it in a laboratory for cancer cells; if they are present, you may need a scan, blood tests or x-rays.

Testicular cancer

Your GP will give you a physical examination. He may send you for an ultrasound. If a lump is present, a biopsy may be taken.

Chapter 3
The treatment options: orthodox medicine

Coping with the diagnosis of cancer, in any form, is one of the major crises that can affect anyone. As we said before, the description of the word *crisis* is a turning point and this is exactly how the situation needs to be treated.

Sometimes there can be language problems; doctors are used to medical jargon and sometimes find it hard to translate it into everyday words. As well as that, doctors are faced with the fear of offering too much hope – unless it can be proven, offering too much hope of a cure is illegal. This, of course, means that they dwell more on the negative side.

Time

Frequently, in a very short time after the diagnosis, the individual has to make instant treatment decisions and a rapid appearance on the surgeon's table. These events are like a roller-coaster and leave the patient without a chance to think, or to come to terms with the situation, and certainly without any real time to make an educated choice. One of my patients was told, 'Of course, you have cancer – we'll remove the breast tomorrow.' The surgeon didn't even discuss the options or let her make a choice!

Experts agree that the earlier cancer is treated, the better chance you have of surviving it. This is because the longer the tumour has to grow, the bigger it gets, the more aggressive it gets and the more likely it is that you will have metastasis – as discussed in the previous chapter. However, this needs to be balanced against your need for time to come to terms with what's happening and to make a decision about the treatment you would prefer. A few days of thinking time is unlikely to make a difference to your treatment unless your cancer is at an extremely advanced stage.

Making a choice

Choice is the critical factor in life. All of us have the chance to choose our option at every point, at all times in our lives. We have both the ability and the right to control our own lives and, when something is considered a life-threatening situation, it is even more important to be able to exercise the option of informed choice. And the choice from the heart is always the inspiration.

In order to make a decision based on fact, it is important to be aware of everything relating to the forms of treatment available. There are many options in orthodox, alternative and complementary treatments. It is also important to understand that choosing to start with one option does not necessarily preclude the benefits and support of the others.

Seeing an oncologist

Most large hospitals have an oncology department, and there are several different ways in which you can see an oncologist or specialist in cancer.

Firstly, your GP may refer you to a local specialist.

Secondly, if you're looking for alternative advice, talk to a naturopath or qualified alternative therapist. Many therapists will have worked with cancer specialists who may be more open-minded, and will be able to refer you to an oncologist who is more sympathetic to alternative methods. I've worked with a number of oncologists who have encouraged patients to control their own diet because it means they'll respond better to orthodox treatment. If there's any conflict in the advice you receive, don't be scared to ask for a second opinion; a second specialist will either give you the comfort factor of confirming the first, or will give you another choice.

Thirdly, you can consult a private specialist, though this of course will need to be paid for, either out of your own pocket or through a private health insurance scheme.

Orthodox medicine

From the orthodox medical point of view, the treatment will consist of surgery, chemotherapy or radiotherapy, or a combination of all or any. These are treatments applied to the person with no individual involvement required. They are done *to* the individual and not *by* the individual. When the statistics are analysed with all types of cancer across the board, the life expectancy is very much the same whether or not these forms of treatment are applied, or whether no treatment is given. The main difference is the quality of life in between.

Some forms of cancer respond well to orthodox treatment and the averages are kept down by conditions such as breast cancer, which has recently been responding well to the drug Tamoxifen and other forms of treatment. What the figures do not show is the long-term outcome, as the treatment has not been going long enough to see how permanent the *cure* is.

Surgery

This is where the tumour itself is removed; you will be given a general anaesthetic before the operation, so you will be asleep during the surgical procedure. Some normal tissue surrounding the tumour may also be removed; this is partly to make sure that all the cancerous cells have been removed, and also to compare the cancer cells with healthy cells. Lymph nodes (special tissues in your immune system that destroy or filter out infections before they pass into the bloodstream) near the tumour may also be removed, to check the spread of any cancer cells lodged in them; any organs in the body already affected by the cancer may also be removed. Reconstructive surgery may also be performed – for example, in the case of a mastectomy.

Surgery is not only performed with a knife. Other forms include:
• *Cryosurgery* – this is where tumours are destroyed by freezing them with liquid nitrogen, applied to the tumour by spray or probe; the freezing-thawing process is repeated, and the body will naturally remove the dead cells. It tends to be used more for skin cancer
• *Chemosurgery* – this is where tumours are destroyed when a chemical is repeatedly applied to their surface. It tends to be used for skin cancer
• *Electrocautery or electrosurgery* – this is where cancer cells are killed by a high-frequency electric current. Again, it tends to be used for skin cancer and also for cancer of the mouth or rectum
• *Laser surgery* – this is where the tumour is destroyed by a laser beam. It is used in cancer of the eye, mouth, throat, oesophagus, cervix and bladder

The side-effects of treatment obviously depend on the kind of surgery under-taken. Minimal surgery has the least side-effects, but major surgery can have knock-on effects both psychologically and physiologically.

In all cases, your body has to cope with the trauma of the operation itself and cope with the anaesthetic; it also has to cope with the healing process after the surgery has been performed. You may feel discomfort and have some bleeding following surgery; the wound can become infected and there may be some swelling (oedema) around the site of the operation.

In the longer term, you may suffer from some nerve pain – a burning sen-sation when nerve-endings that were damaged during the operation grow back. You may also suffer from lymphoedema; this is the build-up of fluid in an area where lymph nodes have been removed causing swelling.

Postural problems can be caused by changes in the body's weight distribution. Surgery – the removal of the tumour – changes your body weight so you need to do compensatory exercises to make up for the change in your balance. Remember that if your body's ability to use energy is decreased, your direct debits will bounce.

Particular problems caused by surgery include:
• With a mastectomy, psychological problems may occur as a woman may feel some of her femininity has been removed
• If the lymph nodes in the armpit (called the axillary nodes) are removed, it will be more painful and also affect your ability to move your arm
• With a colostomy, the whole of the colon is removed; this is the far end of the intestine, but it also absorbs nutrients, so you need to eat greater quantities of the critical nutrients. Obviously, this leads to a lot of wastage

Radiotherapy
Radiotherapy is where the cancer cells are destroyed or their ability to reproduce is prevented by radioactive material. If an abnormal cell that has received radiation tries to divide and reproduce, it fails and dies in the attempt. Normal cells are able to recover from exposure to radiation but this ability decreases with the number of times the cells are exposed to radiation.

The main types of radiotherapy used are:
• *External beam radiation* – this is when radiation from a source outside the body is focused on the area of the body affected by the cancer; the source is

usually an electron beam or a high-energy X-ray. It is painless and you will not need to stay in hospital during your treatment. The treatment does not make you radioactive, so you do not need to avoid other people during your treatment.

• *Internal beam radiation* (also known as a brachytherapy) – this is when radioactive material is placed into the tumour itself and left in place for a while, then removed. Because surgery is involved, you will need to stay in hospital for a short while during the treatment.

Radiotherapy is less invasive than chemotherapy because it is focused on a particular part of the body rather than travelling through the bloodstream. However, it damages good cells as well as bad, so you will always have scans before the radiotherapy to pinpoint the exact location of the tumour – this means the treatment is focused as closely as possibly on the bad cells and minimises the damage to the good cells. The radiographer will mark your skin with ink to show where the radiation needs to be focused.

External beam radiation is usually given over a period of around four to six weeks, for a few minutes each day; the spreading-out of the treatment allows your normal cells to repair themselves. If all the cancer cells are not killed, the tumour may regrow and repeated radiation treatment will not be effective as normal tissues are less able to withstand the effects of further radiation.

Radiotherapy is used for skin cancers; cancers of the mouth, nasal cavity, pharynx and larynx; brain tumours and many gynaecological, lung, and prostate cancers. It is also used in breast cancer, bowel cancer, bladder cancer, Hodgkin's disease, leukaemia, lymphomas, thyroid cancer, childhood cancers, gynaecological and testes tumours.

Side-effects of radiotherapy are usually temporary. They vary from patient to patient and also depend on the dose of radiation you receive and the area of the body which is treated. The most common side-effects include:

• *Radiation nausea* – this tends to be worse just after the treatment. You can ease the effects by sipping ice-cold drinks, avoiding strong-smelling or high-fat foods, and eating small, frequent, well-balanced meals, slowly. Eating a light meal 1-2 hours before the treatment may help

• *Hair loss* – unlike with some drugs, the hair loss will not be all over your body, but only within the area that has received radiation

• *Fatigue* – this is the most common symptom and it may be due to a mixture of the disease itself, the treatment, a lowered blood count, lack of sleep, stress, pain and poor appetite. You need to rest after treatment to give your body a chance to recover; go by how you feel. If sitting or lying down means that you're going to brood on the situation and feel worse, then do something that doesn't require much expenditure of energy but will take your mind off your situation. You may find that several short naps help more than a long rest. Light exercise (such as walking) can also help

• *Blood count changes* – because the radiation damages lymphocytes (white blood cells in your body's immune system that defend your body against invading organisms) in the blood stream and lymph nodes, and your bone marrow cells have been exposed to radiation, certain elements of your blood will be reduced after treatment: particularly white blood cells, lymphocytes and platelets. A low white cell count will make you more susceptible to infections and low platelets mean you're likely to suffer nosebleeds, blood in the urine, heavier periods (for women) and you may bruise easily. This is more marked if you are also receiving chemotherapy

• *Skin reactions* – these include reddening, dryness and crusting and they may take up to six weeks to heal. Try to avoid irritation from clothing, deodorants and perfumes, and leave the area open to the air if you can, though avoid the sun you'll be more likely to burn

• *Mucous membrane reactions* – reddening and soreness (called mucositis) and a plaque-like substance similar to skin crusting may appear. Depending on which membranes are affected, you may have a cough, hoarseness, diarrhoea or abdominal cramps. You're also more likely to suffer from thrush and you may suffer from permanent dryness of the mouth some months after treatment. Try to keep your mouth as clean as possible, using dental floss, a soft toothbrush and mouthwash

• *Scarring* – the tissues in the area treated may be less supple and less resistant to injury or trauma

• *Fertility problems* – if a woman's ovaries or a man's testes are being treated by radiotherapy, there is a risk of infertility and reduced hormone output; your consultant will discuss this with you before treatment is given

Chemotherapy

Chemotherapy is when the tumour is killed by drugs. These can be in tablet form, by direct injection into the bloodstream (intravenous – this can also be via a fluid drip, where a bottle of the drug is hung on a pole, a tube runs from the bottle to the needle in your vein, and the drug drips in at a specified rate) or by intramuscular injection. It's usually given in cycles of treatments, around three to four weeks apart, for a total of four to six months. Between the cycles of treatments, your normal cells will recover but the cancer cells will not.

It's harder for the body to cope with drugs injected directly into the bloodstream as they're not targeted and will affect your whole immune system, killing good as well as bad cells. The longer the treatment goes on, the more support your body needs to cope with it. You'll need extra nutritional support so that your immune system can sandbag the body's functions.

Before you are offered chemotherapy, your doctor will take into account your general condition, the function of your liver and kidneys, and how advanced your tumour is. The amount of drugs you are given depends on your height and weight; you will be given blood and urine tests during your treatment and your chemotherapy dose may be altered between cycles, depending on the results of the tests and how your body reacts to the drugs.

Chemotherapy can be either a single drug or a cocktail of different drugs. A combination drug may contain elements which make other drugs more potent or help to avoid the problem of cancer cells becoming resistant to one particular drug. The drugs either affect the development of the cancer cell, or send it a confusing message that makes it do the wrong thing and destroy itself. The drugs enter the body, kill the abnormal cells (which divide and grow very quickly) and leave the body before they can damage the slower-dividing healthy cells. However, the drugs can affect healthy cells which divide quickly, particularly those in the bone marrow, digestive tract (mouth, oesophagus, stomach and intestines), sexual organs and hair follicles.

The forms of cancer that respond best to chemotherapy include:
• Cancers that have large proportions of dividing cells
• Small tumours (either because they have been detected early or because most of the tumour has already been removed by surgery or radiotherapy)
• Systemic cancers (such as leukaemia and lymphoma)

The main forms of chemotherapy drugs include:
• *Alkylating agents* – these interfere with cell division. They work by cross-linking two components of the cell's DNA, which confuses it so that it destroys itself.

• *Antimetabolites* – these stop the cells metabolising by blocking the formation of *building block* chemical reactions which the cell needs to reproduce itself, either by blocking one of the enzymes involved in cell reproduction or by giving the cell a false DNA building block

• *Vinca alkaloids* (or plant alkaloids) – these are chemicals derived from plants, particularly the periwinkle. They stop the cells dividing by binding to them

• *Antibiotics* – these interact with the cancer cell DNA to break the DNA strand, interfere with enzyme production or bind with the DNA; any of these will stop the cells dividing

• *Hormones* – these give messages which affect cell growth. Steroid hormones are used for prostate, breast, uterus and kidney cancers, and glucocorticoid hormones are used for Hodgkin's disease, lymphoma, leukaemia and myeloma

The side-effects of chemotherapy and their severity differ from person to person; they may also differ in the same person from session to session.

The most common side effects include:

• *Nausea and vomiting* – this tends to be in the first four to twenty-four hours after treatment. You can help ease the effects by sipping ice-cold drinks, avoiding high-fat or strong-smelling foods and eating small, frequent, well-balanced meals slowly. Your doctor may offer you an anti-emetic (anti-sickness) drug

• *Hair loss* – the rate of hair loss varies, as does the amount; you may suffer a little thinning or lose all your hair, including eyebrows and body hair. However, your hair should return after the chemotherapy has finished. At first, it will be baby-fine but when the treatment has finished your hair will grow back as thick – if not thicker – than before. Use a mild shampoo and a soft hair brush, and use a low heat if you use a hairdryer. Avoid hair treatments such as dyeing and perming

• *Bone-marrow depression* – this affects the immune system. If you have a low red blood cell count, you will be anaemic and suffer from tiredness and breathlessness; low white cell count will make you more susceptible to infections (you may feel hot then cold and clammy, and your temperature will rise); and low platelets mean you're likely to suffer nosebleeds, blood in the urine, heavier periods (for women) and may bruise easily. Your blood count will be checked regularly throughout your treatment; but tell your doctor if you have any unexpected bruising, black or bloody bowel movements, feeling of warmth or heat in your arms or legs, or any small red spots under the skin

• *Lack of energy or fatigue* – this is the most common symptom and it may be due to a mixture of the disease itself, the treatment, a lowered blood count, lack of sleep, stress, pain and poor appetite. You need to rest after treatment to give your body a chance to recover. Several short naps may help you more than a longer rest; gentle walking can also help

• *Irregular or missed periods (for women)* – some chemotherapy drugs affect the amount of hormones the ovaries produce; it can bring on the menopause or cause infertility (either temporary or permanent). Your doctor will discuss this with you before treatment

• *Pain* – this may be from damage to nerves (often in the fingers or toes). Tell your doctor where the pain is, how it feels (throbbing, sharp, steady), how strong it is, how long it lasts, whether anything makes it feel better or worse, and what you've taken for it. Your doctor may be able to give you painkillers, or relaxation exercises may help you deal with the pain

• *Constipation* – chemotherapy can cause constipation, especially if you're less active, you're not drinking enough or eating enough fibre. Don't take laxatives without talking to your doctor first; instead, try drinking plenty of fluids (warm or hot drinks are particularly useful), take some gentle exercise, and check with your doctor whether you can increase the amount of fibre in your diet (eg wholemeal bread and cereals, vegetables, fruit and nuts)

• *Diarrhoea* – chemotherapy can cause loose or watery stools. Tell your doctor if it lasts for more than 24 hours or you have any stomach cramps; otherwise, drink plenty of fluids and eat small, frequent meals that are rich in potassium (bananas are a good source). Don't drink very hot or cold fluids and avoid coffee, tea and alcohol. Milk products can make diarrhoea worse; avoid them until the problem has cleared up

• *Sore mouth* – try to keep your mouth as clean as possible, using dental floss, a soft toothbrush and mouthwash. If you have mouth ulcers, your clinic may be able to give you a special mouthwash to help

Overall, medical treatments have improved and are more skilled than they used to be – much more of a rifle shot than a scattergun approach. They are less traumatic for the body than they used to be, but the fact remains that any toxic matter put into your body will affect normal function, and you need to look at supporting your body. A good way of doing this is through alternative and complementary therapies, as we shall see in the next chapter.

Orthodox treatment of the more common types of cancer

Bladder cancer
Surgery
The cancer is cut away through a special thin tube called a cystoscope and a

mild electrical current seals the area. The procedure is called transurethal rescetion. It may need to be repeated every few months as the cancer will tend to come back.

If the cancer has spread into the bladder wall, the part of the bladder that contains the cancer may be removed. If it's too widespread, the whole of your bladder may need to be removed – a procedure known as a cystectomy – and a small section of your bowel will be used to join your urethra (the tube through which you pass water) from your kidneys to the skin of your stomach. This will drain into a small bag attached to the side of your stomach.

The cystectomy will be done under a general anaesthetic – that is, you'll be asleep during the operation – and some of the nearby organs may also need to be removed. In men, these are the prostate gland and part of the urethra; in women, the urethra, front wall of the vagina, womb, fallopian tubes and ovaries may be removed.

Radiotherapy

A radiation beam will be focused on the part of your body affected by cancer. Before the treatment begins, you will have scans and x-rays so that the surgeons can pinpoint the exact location of the cancer and mark the relevant area on your skin with ink.

Chemotherapy

For superficial bladder cancer, where only the lining of the bladder is affected, you may be offered intravesical chemotherapy. This is where anti-cancer drugs are placed directly into your bladder through a thin tube called a catheter. You hold the drugs in your bladder for an hour before emptying it. The treatment is usually given once a week for several weeks, following surgery.

For invasive bladder cancer, where the whole of the bladder is affected and the cancer has spread to other organs or the lymph nodes, anti-cancer drugs will be injected into your veins or you may be able to take the medication orally.

Bowel cancer

Surgery

Around 80 per cent of people with bowel cancer have surgery. A bowel resection is where the surgeon removes the area of diseased tissue and a small amount of the surrounding tissue; he or she will then join the remaining sections of the bowel together or will give you a colostomy, where the end of the bowel is brought to the surface of the skin on the abdomen so that waste can be removed.

Radiotherapy

If surgery isn't possible, or if the surgeon wants to shrink the tumour before surgery, you may be offered radiotherapy.

In external beam radiation, a radiation beam will be focused on the part of your body affected by cancer to destroy any remaining cancer cells. Before the treatment begins, you will have scans and x-rays so that the surgeons can pinpoint the exact location of the cancer and mark the relevant area on your skin with ink

With internal beam radiation (also known as brachytherapy), the surgeon will place a small pellet of radioactive material into the lump. The procedure is done under anaesthetic and you will need a short stay in hospital.

Chemotherapy

This is usually used in conjunction with surgery. Anti-cancer drugs are injected into your veins to kill the cells or stop them multiplying.

Brain cancer

The treatment offered depends on the size, location and type of tumour.

Surgery

This is the most common treatment and is done under a general anaesthetic. The surgeon will make an opening in your skull (a craniotomy) and remove as much of the tumour as possible. This may also help to relieve symptoms caused by the build-up of pressure in the skull.

Radiotherapy

If only part of the tumour can be removed, or surgery is not possible, you may be given radiotherapy.

In external beam radiation, a radiation beam will be focused on the part of your body affected by cancer to destroy any remaining cancer cells. Before the treatment, you will have scans and x-rays so the surgeons can pinpoint the exact location of the cancer and mark the relevant area on your skin with ink.

With internal beam radiation (also known as brachytherapy or interstitial radiotherapy), the surgeon places a small pellet of radioactive material into the lump. This is done under anaesthetic and you will need a short stay in hospital.

Chemotherapy

Because the brain is protected by thin membranes that filter drugs from the bloodstream, some anti-cancer drugs are not effective. However, other anti-cancer drugs have been shown to work and may be available either orally or injected into your veins.

Breast cancer

The treatment depends on the age of the woman and the size of the tumour.

Surgery

A *lumpectomy* is where the lump itself and some of the surrounding tissue is removed – not the whole breast. It is almost always followed by radiotherapy. A *partial or segmental mastectomy* is where the lump and up to a quarter of the breast is removed; as with a lumpectomy, it is almost always followed by radiotherapy.

A *mastectomy* is where the whole breast is removed. The lymph nodes under your armpit and some of your chest muscle (pectoral) may be removed, although this is less common nowadays as surgical techniques have improved.

You may be offered reconstructive surgery; this could take the form of a breast implant or *autologous reconstruction*, where part of your abdomen is used to build a mould that looks like a normal breast. An alternative is a prosthesis or false breast that can be fitted into a bra.

Radiotherapy

In external beam radiation, a radiation beam will be focused on the part of your body affected by cancer to destroy any remaining cancer cells. Before the treatment begins, you will have scans and x-rays so that the surgeons can pinpoint the exact location of the cancer and mark the relevant area on your skin with ink.

With internal beam radiation (also known brachytherapy), the surgeon will place a radioactive iridium wire into the breast tissue; it is left in place for a few days and then removed. The procedure is done under anaesthetic and you will need a short stay in hospital.

Chemotherapy

Anti-cancer drugs will be injected into your veins or you may be able to take the medication orally.

Hormone drugs

Breast cancers are fed by oestrogen, a hormone produced by your ovaries. In hormone treatment, you will be given a drug that will attach itself to the receptors on the cancer cells so that oestrogen can't affect them. The most commonly used drug is Tamoxifen. It is taken daily as a tablet for five years following surgery, although the *Cancer Research Campaign* and *Imperial Cancer Fund* are running a trial to see if it can also prevent breast cancer in women who are at a high risk of developing it.

Cervical cancer

Surgery

If the changes in the cells are pre-cancerous, the doctor may use cryosurgery (freezing), cauterisation (burning) or laser surgery to destroy the abnormal cells without harming normal cells. Another method is the cone biopsy where tissue is removed surgically.

If the cancer is confined to the cervix, the surgeon may be able to remove the cancer but leave the womb and ovaries; if it has spread, you may need a hysterectomy (the surgical removal of your womb).

Radiotherapy

In external beam radiation, a radiation beam will be focused on the part of your body affected by cancer to destroy any remaining cancer cells. Before the treatment begins, you will have scans and x-rays so that the surgeons can pinpoint the exact location of the cancer and mark the relevant area on your skin with ink.

With internal beam radiation (also known as brachytherapy), the surgeon will place a small pellet of radioactive material into the vagina; it is left in place for a few days and then removed. The procedure is done under anaesthetic and you will need a short stay in hospital.

Chemotherapy

At the moment, this tends to be used only for advanced or recurrent cases of cervical cancer.

Lung cancer

The treatment depends on the type of cancer.

For non-small lung cell cancer (NSCLC):

Surgery

This is only performed when the cancer is found at an early stage. The surgeon may remove a small part of your lung (known as a segmentectomy or wedge resection), an entire section (a lobectomy) or the entire lung (pneumonectomy). The operation is done under a general anaesthetic and you will need to stay in hospital for a couple of weeks afterwards. Pain management after surgery is important because you will need to be able to cough and breathe deeply to avoid infection in the remaining part of your lungs.

Radiotherapy

In external beam radiation, a radiation beam will be focused on the part of your body affected by cancer to destroy any remaining cancer cells. Before the treatment begins, you will have scans and x-rays so that the surgeons can pinpoint the exact location of the cancer and mark the relevant area on your skin with ink.

With internal beam radiation (also known as brachytherapy), the surgeon will place a small pellet of radioactive material into the tumour or the airways next to the tumour for a short period, and then remove it.

Chemotherapy

Anti-cancer drugs will be injected into your veins or medication may be given orally. It may be before surgery, to shrink the tumour, or afterwards.

For small lung cell cancer (SCLC):

Chemotherapy

Chemotherapy is the main treatment of small lung cell cancer because there are likely to be undetected cancer cells scattered through your body, and SCLC is not usually suitable for surgery. Anti-cancer drugs will be injected into your veins or you may be able to take the medication orally.

Lymphoma cancer

Watchful waiting

Your specialist may suggest no treatment other than regular check-ups to ensure that the position hasn't changed. This is known as watchful waiting. If the disease becomes rapidly progressive or there's a failure of bone marrow, treatment will be started.

Radiotherapy

In external beam radiation, a radiation beam will be focused on the part of your body affected by cancer to destroy any remaining cancer cells. Before treatment, you will have scans and x-rays so that surgeons can pinpoint the exact location of the cancer and mark the relevant area on your skin.

Chemotherapy

Anti-cancer drugs will be injected into your veins or you may be able to take the medication orally. If there are cancer cells in your spinal fluid, the drugs may be injected directly into your spinal fluid.

Interferon

Interferon is a hormone-like substance produced by your white blood cells to help your immune system fight infections. Interferon can shrink tumours or prolong remission and is commonly given after chemotherapy.

Prostate cancer

Watchful waiting

Some prostate cancers grow slowly and may not cause clinical problems, so your specialist may suggest no treatment other than regular check-ups to ensure that the position hasn't changed. This is known as watchful waiting.

Surgery

If your prostate cancer is growing quickly and you are relatively young, your specialist may suggest a prostatectomy; this is the surgical removal of the prostate gland and some of the surrounding tissue, and is done under a general anaesthetic. You will need a catheter – a plastic tube – to drain your bladder of urine for about three weeks, until your urethra (the tube that passes water from your bladder to your penis) has healed.

Radiotherapy

If the cancer is in the prostate gland only, you may be offered radiotherapy as an alternative to surgery.

In external beam radiation, a radiation beam will be focused on the part of your body affected by cancer to destroy any remaining cancer cells. Before the treatment begins, you will have scans and x-rays so that the surgeons can pinpoint the exact location of the cancer and mark the relevant area on your skin with ink.

With internal beam radiation (also known as brachytherapy), the surgeon will place a small pellet of radioactive material into your prostate gland. This may be permanent (low-dose) or it may be removed after a few minutes (high dose) and repeated the next day. The procedure is done under anaesthetic and you will need a short stay in hospital.

Chemotherapy

Chemotherapy is rarely used as a treatment for prostate cancer, except to relieve pain, because the tumours tend to be slow-growing and the chemotherapy drugs have not been very successful in treating them.

Hormone therapy

Hormone therapy (depriving the growth of the hormone testosterone) can make the growth shrink. It is often used if the cancer has spread outside the prostate gland to your bones. The main type of hormone treatment is known as LHRH-agonist; it's an injection given monthly or every three months into your abdomen, and the drugs stop your testes producing testosterone.

Skin cancer

Surgery

The surgeon will remove the melanoma and some normal tissue around it to make sure the cancer cells are removed. Some of your lymph nodes may also be removed.

Chemotherapy

If the cancer has spread to other parts of the body, chemotherapy may be offered. Anti-cancer drugs will be injected into your veins or you may be able to take the medication orally

Testicular cancer

Surgery

The surgeon will remove your testicle – this is known as an orchiectomy

Chemotherapy

Anti-cancer drugs will be injected into your veins or you may be able to take the medication orally

Side-effects of orthodox treatment for the more common types of cancer

As well as the general side-effects mentioned previously (see page 50), you may suffer from side-effects specific to your particular cancer

Bladder cancer

Surgery

• You may feel discomfort and have some bleeding following surgery

• Women whose wombs have to be removed will no longer be able to have children. Your vagina will be narrower and shorter so you may experience difficulties with sexual intercourse.

• Men may become impotent; if your prostate gland is removed, you will not longer be able to produce semen and will not be able to ejaculate.

• Postural problems can be caused by the changes in the body's weight distribution

Radiotherapy

• You may experience skin changes similar to sunburn
• You may suffer from nausea, bladder irritation, diarrhoea and fatigue

Chemotherapy

• If you have intravesical chemotherapy, your bladder may be irritated and you may have a burning sensation in your bladder
• You may suffer from nausea, vomiting, hair loss, mouth sores
• If your bone marrow cells are affected, you may be more likely to pick up infections, bleed or bruise after minor cuts, and have a lowered blood count that will cause you to feel breathless and tired

Bowel cancer

Surgery

• Your bowel movements may be more liquid and you may be unable to eat some foods
• You may have problems urinating or having sexual intercourse

Radiotherapy

• You may experience skin changes similar to sunburn
• You may suffer from nausea, diarrhoea and fatigue

Chemotherapy

• You may suffer from nausea, vomiting, hair loss, mouth sores, soreness of the hands and feet and have a strange taste in your mouth
• Some drugs may cause you to become infertile
• Women may find that their periods stop until the treatment is completed

Brain cancer

Surgery

• You may suffer from some swelling (oedema) around the site of the operation; this can cause weakness, personality changes, co-ordination problems and difficulty in talking or thinking

Radiotherapy

• You may experience skin changes similar to sunburn – keep out of the sun as your skin will be more sensitive, and wear a hat
• If the radiotherapy damages and kills normal brain tissue, you may have headaches, memory loss or fits months after the treatment

Chemotherapy

• You may suffer from nausea, vomiting, hair loss, mouth sores
• Some drugs can cause kidney damage, tingling in your fingers and ringing in your ears
• If your bone marrow cells are affected, you may be more likely to pick up infections, bleed or bruise after minor cuts, and have a lowered blood count that will cause you to feel breathless and tired

Breast cancer

Surgery

• You may suffer from lymphoedema – accumulation of fluid which causes swelling in your upper arms, hands and fingers
• The wound may become infected, or blood (a haematoma) or clear fluid (sermona) may accumulate in the wound

• You may have temporary limitation in the movement of your arm and shoulder

Radiotherapy
• You may experience skin changes similar to sunburn – keep out of the sun as your skin will be more sensitive
• As with surgery, radiotherapy can cause lymphoedema if your lymph nodes under your armpit have been treated

Chemotherapy
• You may suffer from nausea, vomiting, hair loss, mouth sores
• If your bone marrow cells are affected, you may be more likely to pick up infections, bleed or bruise after minor cuts, and have a lowered blood count that will cause you to feel breathless and tired
• Some particular drugs can cause cystitis, diarrhoea and turn your urine red (temporarily)

Hormonal treatments
You may notice changes in your menstrual cycle or menopausal symptoms such as hot flushes, nausea and indigestion

Cervical cancer
Surgery
• Side-effects are rare but there is a risk of bleeding and infection after the operation. You may have temporary problems with the function of your bowel and bladder

• If your ovaries are removed, you will be infertile

Radiotherapy
• You may experience skin changes similar to sunburn
• You may suffer from diarrhoea and nausea
• You may suffer from premature menopause
• You may find sexual intercourse painful if your vagina shrinks and loses its elasticity
• If your ovaries are affected, you will be infertile

Chemotherapy
• You may suffer from nausea, vomiting, hair loss, mouth sores
• If your bone marrow cells are affected, you may be more likely to pick up infections, bleed or bruise after minor cuts, and have a lowered blood count that will cause you to feel breathless and tired
• Some drugs can cause kidney damage, tingling in your fingers and ringing in your ears

Lung cancer

Surgery
• You may suffer from shortness of breath, particularly if you have emphysema or chronic bronchitis
• It can take up to 6 months to recover from surgery

Radiotherapy
• You may experience skin changes similar to sunburn
• You may feel tired and have a sore or dry throat

- You may be stiff in the chest or shoulder
- Rib movement and mobility may be uncomfortable

Chemotherapy
- You may suffer from nausea, vomiting, hair loss, mouth sores
- If your bone marrow cells are affected, you may be more likely to pick up infections, bleed or bruise after minor cuts, and have a lowered blood count that will cause you to feel breathless and tired

Lymphoma cancer

Radiotherapy
- You may experience skin changes similar to sunburn
- You may feel tired or suffer from nausea, diarrhoea and vomiting

Chemotherapy
- You may suffer from nausea, vomiting, hair loss, mouth sores.
- If your bone marrow cells are affected, you may be more likely to pick up infections, bleed or bruise after minor cuts, and have a lowered blood count that will cause you to feel breathless and tired

Interferon
- You may suffer from tiredness, fever, chills, headaches, muscle and joint aches and mood changes

Prostate cancer

Surgery
- 70 per cent of men suffer from impotence afterwards

• 40 per cent of men suffer from incontinence afterwards

Radiotherapy
• Diarrhoea
• Cystitis
• 30–40 per cent of men suffer from impotence afterwards

Hormone therapy
• Impotence
• Hot flushes
• Swelling of the breast area (rare)

Skin cancer
Surgery
• Scar formation
• You may suffer from lymphoedema – accumulation of fluid which causes swelling in your upper arms, hands and fingers

Testicular cancer
Surgery
If lymph nodes are removed, it may affect the nerves involved in ejaculation.

Chapter 4
The treatment options: alternative and complementary medicine

Alternative and complementary therapies

There is a wide range of alternative and complementary therapies available.

Alternative therapies are used instead of conventional medical treatment and often involve a complete change in philosophy. They can be used very effectively, especially by practitioners who use them to restore normal function rather than merely treating the symptoms.

Complementary therapies aim to help you feel better. They work well with either the alternative or the traditional approach, and several different complementary therapies can be used together. Complementary therapies are particularly good at helping to combat stress – which affects our immune systems – and can also help to manage pain and deal with side-effects of orthodox treatment.

Some orthodox practitioners believe that complementary therapies in particular have only a placebo effect – that is, similar to a pill made of sugar that does no harm but also doesn't have any particular power to cure. However, placebos can be a very effective form of treatment, because they give the patient confidence. Complementary and alternative practitioners tend to have more time to talk to patients, which makes patients feel more confident and believe in the treatment; and belief is a major part of the healing process.

With all alternative and complementary therapies, you need to make sure that your practitioner is qualified. A list of organisations which can help you find a qualified practitioner is in Appendix 1.

Alternative therapies

Alternatives include extremely radical diet and supplementary applications such as the Gerson system – a very restrictive, stringent diet which uses coffee enemas, working on the principle that absorbing caffeine through the intestine will help the body. However, neither enemas nor caffeine are natural for the body; although the system works for some people, caffeine is a toxin and I do not recommend it.

Hydrotherapeutic and colonic irrigation enema techniques have been used extensively in selected practices and have helped many people to achieve very good results. This system is a treatment of the condition targeted very carefully at a problem called cancer, and I would view this as an alternative form of esoteric medicine.

Naturopathy

Naturopaths have for many years offered people an alternative approach to cancer, although it can also be seen as complementary medicine. Naturopathy is an approach rather than a cure or a treatment, because it is illegal for unregistered practitioners to treat cancer.

The approach is basically a combination of nutrition supplementation, hydrotherapy and exercise aimed at restoring the body's normal function rather than treating the condition. The diet needs to start with cutting out anything that has low nutritional values, such as refined and highly processed foods, alcohol and stimulants. Thirty or forty years ago, people who refused treatment on religious grounds were advised to fast for five or six weeks, or use a monodiet such as grapes. The body therefore uses less energy in digestion of food and elimination of waste products, which leaves more energy in the bank account, which can then be used as a direct debit for healing. With complete fasting, all energy goes into elimination and repair; and as elimination starts, the healing process begins.

I believe that you need to have a balanced diet, containing organic food; you also need to eat regularly and have the right mental attitude towards eating. It's important that you make your own choice, to take as radical or as conservative a path as you want – fasting, a monodiet or having a choice of food. You will however need to supplement your diet with vitamins; sadly, even organic food is deficient in vitamins, as we shall see in Chapter 5.

Many people have achieved remarkable results themselves, by following the advice they have been given, to re-create health and enable the body to recover the function of its immune system and its general metabolism to deal with the problems from an internal and self-empowered point of view. One of my patients, a lady of 55, had liver cancer diagnosed seven weeks previously; she had read an article on the treatment I had given Helen Rollason and started some of the dietary advice prior to consulting me. She refused chemotherapy as in 1998 she had a lumpectomy and then a full mastectomy in 1991. After the mastectomy she had a diagnosis of bone cancer. She started on the organic targeted diet and took the food state vitamins and minerals, pre-biotic and pro-biotic, and the enhanced water; she has made steady and consistent progress ever since. She is now living a normal life and maintains a sensible balanced or organic diet and is taking walking holidays. She wrote to me last year, telling me how much she had enjoyed Christmas, which she didn't expect to be around for.

Another patient had breast cancer diagnosed in October 1996. She had a lumpectomy, lymphectomy, chemotherapy and radiotherapy; nine months later, she found a rash on the scar, and three months later cancer was diagnosed in her lymphatic system. She had a radical mastectomy but the rash returned and did not respond to chemotherapy.

She had further lumps and skin tissue removed, and yet more chemotherapy, the last treatment being in December 1998. When she saw me, I suggested dietary changes; when I examined her in May 1999 she was feeling extremely well and all conditions in relation to carcinogenic activity had improved – she was told by her oncologist that her cancer was in remission.

Within the naturopathic approach, the individual is responsible for making all the necessary changes in lifestyle and mental attitude and is empowering himself or herself to deal with the problem internally, not receiving treatment or applied chemical therapy.

The major problem resulting from this approach has been that, for many years, naturopaths and similar practitioners have been unable to obtain co-operation between themselves and orthodox medicine and people have been given a black or white choice – orthodox or alternative medicine only. This has not made it easy for the individual to make a decision in such a difficult situation. Nowadays, there is a growing awareness in orthodox medicine of the role played by positive lifestyle management and there is growing co-operation between practitioners of different types of treatment.

All the complementary therapies are best used as a back-up to orthodox or alternative treatments. However, they only deal with part of the equation of rebalancing the body – nutritional, structural or emotional, so they are not fully effective without the back-up of the other parts of the equation.

Complementary therapy – acupuncture

Acupuncture is a system of healing first recorded in China and Japan around 4,500 years ago. In common with naturopathy, it is based on the belief that health is dependent on the body's motivating energy moving freely and being balanced. There are around 500 recognised acupuncture points on the body, though they don't necessarily lie near the part of the body being treated – for example, headaches can be treated on points in the feet or the hands.

In traditional acupuncture, needles are inserted into the appropriate point of your body and manipulated. The needles are left in place for up to 20 minutes and you may feel a slight tingling – though it doesn't actually hurt and you shouldn't feel the needles going in. Some practitioners burn herbs near the acupuncture points; this is known as *moxibustion.*

Over thousands of years, many people have used acupuncture as a means of helping to restore the balance of the body's energies and from early Chinese history it has been used as a successful aid to the body, rebalancing itself and stimulating function and the recreation of health from within. It is frequently used nowadays in conjunction with orthodox medical treatment. It's particularly good for helping you to relax and to deal with side-effects of orthodox treatment, including:

• Constipation
• Diarrhoea
• Fatigue
• Pain

Complementary therapy – Alexander Technique

The Alexander Technique is a practical method developed by Australian actor FM Alexander in the late 1800s for improving posture and movement. It focuses on the relationship between your head, neck and torso; when these are properly aligned, your head will lift upwards and release the neck and spine, improving overall muscular function and letting you move your whole body in a harmonious way. The technique teaches you to use the appropriate amount of effort for a particular activity, giving you more energy for all your activities.

It's taught one-to-one by a qualified teacher; you'll need around 30 lessons of 30-40 minutes to learn the technique thoroughly. It helps with structural rebalancing but needs to be backed up by nutritional and emotional rebalancing as well.

It also encourages conscious awareness, a great help in living in the present. It's particularly good for helping you to relax and to deal with side-effects of orthodox treatment, including:

• Abdominal cramps

• Fatigue

• Pain

Complementary therapy – Aromatherapy

Aromatherapy uses essential oils, made from plant extracts; they're very strong, so you should always dilute them in a carrier oil before using in the bath, in massage or in a burner or steam inhaler. The scent of the essential oils is conveyed by the olfactory nerve to areas of the brain that can influence emotions and hormonal response; the oils are also absorbed through the skin during a massage or in a bath, and are carried by body fluids to the nervous and muscular systems.

It's particularly good for helping you to relax and deal with side-effects of orthodox treatment, including:

• Abdominal cramps

• Constipation

• Cough

• Diarrhoea

• Fatigue

- Mouth sores
- Nausea and vomiting
- Oedema
- Pain
- Skin reactions – reddening, dryness and crusting
- Thrush

Complementary therapy – Bach flower remedies

Flower Remedies are based on the work of Dr Edward Bach in the late 1920s; 38 different flower remedies cover every state of mind, either on their own or with up to six of them mixed together. The remedies are used to treat the whole person and their emotional states, rather than physical symptoms, and are selected according to your personality and your emotional state. Dr Bach believed that there were seven major groups of emotional states: fear, uncertainty, lack of interest in your present circumstances, loneliness, over-sensitivity, despondency and too much concern for the welfare of others. The theory is that the remedies restore harmony to the mind and therefore allow the body to heal itself. The flower remedies are made by floating flowers on clear spring water in sunlight; when the water has been impregnated with the healing properties of the flower, it is preserved in brandy. You then take two drops in a glass of pure mineral water.

Bach flower remedies are best used to help you cope with stress and fear; they can also help to deal with fatigue.

Complementary therapy – Colour therapy

Colour therapy is based on ancient systems of using colour and light for healing and on modern colour psychology. The idea behind it is that colour is a vibrational energy which affects personality and behaviour.

By introducing certain colours into clothing, the environment, food and drink or by visualisations, breathing or coloured light treatments, a colour therapist can restore harmony. This is very good for helping to relieve stress and promote relaxation; it can also help you deal with side-effects of orthodox treatment, including:

- Abdominal cramps
- Constipation
- Diarrhoea
- Fatigue
- Mouth sores
- Pain

Complementary therapy – Healing (hands on or off)

Healing – an art which has been used for years under different names – is also frequently used to help people who have cancer in its many forms. Healing is something which cannot be categorised by scientific terms, but thousands of people have been helped and achieved some wonderful results with all forms of problems, including cancer. As with all things, healing is something which one has to consider and learn as much about as possible and then make a choice as appropriate.

Healing is a process of channelling energy through yourself and helping to transfer it to another individual, to open them up to receive the healing life-energy, which balances and re-energises their body so that normal functions start to recur. I've heard of many people who have visited a healer and felt heat or cold travelling down their body, and then discovered that their tumour had become benign.

Healing instils confidence and belief in the process, and helps with the mind state. It can work with almost any other complementary therapy. Some healers are hands-on – that is, they actually touch the body; others use a hands-off approach, where their hands are just above the body; and yet more healers choose a remote approach, where they concentrate their energy on someone who may be across the other side of the country.

It's very good for helping to relieve stress and promote relaxation; it can also help you deal with side-effects of orthodox treatment, including:
- Abdominal cramps
- Fatigue
- Pain

Complementary therapy – Herbalism

Herbalism is the use of plant remedies to treat disease. *The National Institute of Medical Herbalists* says that it is the most widely practised form of medicine worldwide and is the oldest form of medicine known. Treatments can be in the form of tinctures, syrups, capsules and creams, and may also include advice about diet and lifestyle. The prescribed remedy will nourish the parts of the body that have become weakened, restoring the balance of the body and letting it heal itself. Whereas pharmaceutical drugs are based on synthetic versions of single active plant constituents, herbal drugs are extracts from a part of the whole plant, which contain many more active constituents; they are therefore more balanced.

It can also help you deal with anxiety and stress and the side-effects of orthodox treatment, including:
- Abdominal cramps
- Constipation
- Cough
- Diarrhoea
- Fatigue

- Nausea and vomiting
- Oedema
- Pain
- Skin reactions – reddening, dryness and crusting
- Thrush

Complementary therapy – Homeopathy

Homeopathy is a system of medicine developed by the nineteenth-century doctor Samual Hahnemann, where like is treated with like. It uses the Law of Similars, which states, 'that which makes sick shall heal.' This means that an illness, caused by too much of a substance, and the symptoms can be cured by a small dose of the substance, which will make the body heal itself. *Homoios* in Greek means similar and *pathos* means disease or suffering.

The remedies – derived from plants, minerals and metals – are made by dilution and succussion (vigorous shaking) in a solution of alcohol and water; the strength is indicated by numbers and letters, e.g. 12X means that the remedy has been diluted by a factor of ten, 12 times in a row, to produce a dilution of 1 part in a trillion. The more diluted the remedies are, the more *potentised* they are said to be. Homeopaths ascribe the therapeutic action of their remedies to an *essence*, *memory* or *energy imprint* that can mobilise the body's *vital forces*, although traditional medicine attributes its success to coincidence or the placebo effect. Having said that, a review in *The Lancet* in 1997 of double-blind and randomised placebo-controlled clinical trials concluded that the clinical effects of homeopathic medicines had a 2.45 times greater effect than the placebo.

It can also help you deal with anxiety and stress and the side-effects of orthodox treatment, including:

- Abdominal cramps
- Constipation
- Coughing
- Diarrhoea
- Fatigue
- Mouth dryness
- Mouth sores
- Nausea and vomiting
- Oedema
- Pain
- Skin reactions – reddening, dryness and crusting
- Thrush

Complementary therapy – Kinesiology

Kinesiology is derived from chiropractic, acupuncture and nutrition; the theory is that various muscles are associated with specific organs and glands, and weakness in a muscle can signal a problem elsewhere in the body. The aim of kinesiology is to restore postural balance, correct impaired gait, improve the range of motion and restore normal neuromuscular function.

The practitioner will give you tests to see if various muscles can hold a given position against manual pressure. If a muscle can, then it is *fixed*, *strong*, or *locked*, whereas a muscle that gives way immediately is *weak* or *unlocked*.

Treatments may include deep massage, joint manipulation and realignment, cranial therapy (adjustment of the bones that, fused together, make up the skull) and meridian therapy.

Kinesiology can help you relax and is good for pain relief.

Complementary therapy – Magnetic therapy

Magnetic therapy is used for pain relief, primarily in joints and muscles. Small magnetic discs generating a field of 350 to 500 gauss – around 10 times the strength of a refrigerator magnet – are taped to the body over the painful areas. Some practitioners use magnetic beds or blankets, which produce a much stronger field to compensate for their greater distance from the skin. Treatments can last for between a couple of minutes and several days. The idea behind it is that the magnet affects the nervous system, which depends on electrical charges to deliver its signals; magnets may also exert a pull on charged particles within bodily fluids, promoting the flow of blood, boosting levels of oxygen and nutrients, and ultimately relieving pain. They are also thought to be good for stress.

Complementary therapy – Massage

Massage is known to increase the circulation of blood because of the rhythmically applied manual pressure and movement; the stimulation of nerve receptors causes the blood vessels to dilate, which also facilitates blood flow. The oxygen capacity of the blood can increase 10–15 per cent after massage.

It also improves the flow of lymph, which carries impurities and waste away from the tissues; the movement of lymph depends on muscle contractions which is aided by massage.

Massage can help balance muscles by loosening contracted, shortened muscles and stimulating weak muscles, which helps posture and promotes more efficient movement. It can also either stimulate or soothe the nerve endings, depending on what you want from the massage. It's particularly good for relieving stress, constipation, headaches, joint pain and stiffness.

If you are using orthodox therapy to treat cancer, your doctor may be able to give you some guidelines for massage – for example, if there are some areas which should not be massaged or others where only a gentle, stroking touch should be used. Side-effects which can be helped by massage include:

• Abdominal cramps

• Constipation

• Fatigue

• Oedema

• Pain

Complementary therapy – Reflexology

Reflexology has been practised for thousands of years, including by the early Indian, Chinese and Egyptian peoples.

An American surgeon, Dr William Fitzgerald, noted that pressure on specific parts of the body could have an anaesthetising effect on a related area. He divided the body into ten equal and vertical zones, ending in the fingers and toes; pressure on one part of a zone affected everything else within the zone. His theory was further developed in the 1930s by Eunice Ingham, who saw that congestion or tension in any part of the foot mirrors congestion or tension in a corresponding part of the body.

A reflexologist uses his or her hands to apply gentle pressure to the feet, detecting imbalances and working on these points to release blockages and restore the free flow of energy to the whole body. Tensions are eased, and circulation and elimination is improved. Reflexology can help you deal with anxiety and stress and the side-effects of orthodox treatment, including:

• Abdominal cramps

• Constipation

• Cough

• Nausea and vomiting

• Pain

Complementary therapy – Reiki

Reiki is a Japanese word meaning *universal life force energy*. The therapy is a system of natural healing which is believed to have spread through China, Tibet and India several thousand years ago, and was rediscovered by Dr Mikao Usui, a Christian theologian working in Tibet in the late nineteenth century. It is based on using the energy around us and on five affirmations which basically tell us to live in the present.

The practitioner places his or her hands non-intrusively on your body in a sequence of positions which cover the whole body; the positions are each held for several minutes and a full treatment takes between an hour and an hour and a half. There is no massage or manipulation, but you may feel heat, tingling, coolness or throbbing under the practitioner's hands as the energy flows to the source of the problem. It can also help you deal with anxiety and stress and the side-effects of orthodox treatment, including:

• Abdominal cramps

• Fatigue

• Pain

Complementary therapy – Yoga

Yoga is a system of personal development that was developed in India around five thousand years ago. It works as a combination of physical postures, breathing exercises and positive thinking or meditation – *yoga* is the *Sanskrit* word for union – to train the mind and body. It can be done by anyone of any age or ability and is usually taught in classes of between 45 minutes and an hour, though once you've learned the postures you can practice them at home. It's recommended that you practice at least part of the routine every day.

Asanas are postures (slow, physical movements interspersed with still positions) which stretch and tone muscles, joints, the spine and the entire skeleton. You'll repeat the postures up to three times, though some will only be done once. Asanas also work on your internal organs, glands and nerves and release physical and mental tension; they follow a specific order to balance the muscle groups. *Pranayama* or breathing exercises revitalise the body and help to control the mind, which in turn can make you feel calm and refreshed; the practise of positive thinking or meditation gives increased clarity, mental power and concentration. It's particularly good for helping you deal with fatigue and stress when fighting cancer.

The approach of treatment

As we have seen above, there are many options in the complementary and alternative approaches to health and to treatment. A critical factor in looking for something which changes the potential result for the individual is whether the approach is trying to treat the symptom or remove the cause. Symptom treatment can be very effective in the short term, but long-term problems frequently return and there are often unpleasant side-effects to the treatment itself.

Cause-removal techniques require a total involvement from the patient, and a change in lifestyle and mental approach – that is, empowering themselves to let the body do that for which it is designed. Only nature heals.

As previously mentioned, in the past there has been no co-operation, in most cases, between alternative and orthodox therapists, and even strong disagreements on both sides. I believe that there is a huge area of potential co-operation that can change the quality of life and the potential results for anybody who has a problem with cancer. This process is now beginning to come about.

Avoiding side-effects

The side-effects of chemotherapy and radiotherapy listed above are well known: but what is not generally known is that, through the application of basic naturopathic principles and the use of the correct choice of nutritional supplements, these side-effects can be dramatically reduced and in some cases even removed.

By following a particular approach to nutrition and lifestyle, many people have had hair loss dramatically reduced, their skin coloration maintained as normal and sickness and distress kept to an absolute minimal level. One of my patients, a lady of 55, saw me in January 1999, having had a history of two previous sessions of chemotherapy for ovarian cancer which had been treated surgically followed by the presence of secondaries in the liver. She undertook a balanced organic diet, used the pre-biotic and pro-biotic food state vitamins and minerals and the enhanced water, as well as a food state-based booster product which had fructoligosaccharides to help with the basic chemical energy.

This, coupled with her gentle and increasing exercise program, meant that during her chemotherapy she had no hair loss, only one day's nausea and responded much better than expected. She is now maintaining balanced nutrition with the nutritional formula and an organically based regular dietary intake. She has needed no further treatment since and was clear at the last scan.

Naturopaths believe that by giving the body what it needs to function naturally, it will begin to function effectively; it follows that by doing the same thing, even during an invasive attack such as chemotherapy, the body is much better able to cope with the imbalance which the treatment creates while undertaking the specific task for which it has been designed.

One of the major problems of chemotherapy is the damage to the immune system. At the same time as dealing with the cancer cells, it is essential that the immune system should be supported by every means possible to encourage nature to do its wonderful work.

Re-creation of health

The same approach – that of re-empowering the body, to get its immune system functioning once more and to enable health to be re-created – is used if people do not wish to have orthodox treatment and is also hugely effective in supporting alternative and complementary medicine, where people take this as their preferred method of treatment.

I believe that it is wrong to deny anyone the ability to choose to take control over the re-creation of health – their health – rather than just accept the treatment of cancer. In the past, naturopaths tended to feel that orthodox approaches are unnatural and totally against their beliefs to regaining health rather than treating symptoms. However, I feel there should be a recognition of the fact that the body is such a wonderful organism that, with the right help and support, many forms of external attack and chemical treatments can still be used and supported by applying the basic principles of re-creation of health.

In recent months, I have worked with many people who have chosen to use the nutritional and supplemental approach. They have all opted for different types of treatment – including radiotherapy, chemotherapy, surgery or a combination of these treatments, or not having any specific treatment at all. In all cases, the outcome has been remarkable. Apart from the side-effects being reduced, the treatment has been more effective at removing the symptoms and the duration of the treatment has been shorter. What the body can achieve with the help of the individual is an endless wonder.

The most significant factor in relation to using the re-creation of health approach, as either an alternative or a supportive part of every individual's efforts to regain health rather than to treat cancer, is that once the immediate crisis is past, the individual has already taken the necessary steps to dramatically reduce the chances of a reoccurrence of cancer. This is because where health is being created, disease *per se* is always much less liable to occur, and the body can develop and maintain a strong, effective immune system.

The ideal approach

My view is that when someone has been given a diagnosis of cancer there should be a full information service available, to put on the table all the options which can be chosen, how they work individually, how they can work together and what kind of commitment they need from the individual. Once this table of choice has been laid out, they can then select which combination of these various approaches they feel comfortable with, and can confidently pursue a positive physical and mental approach.

The benefits of complementary therapies mentioned previously cannot be underestimated in relation to supporting the naturopathic health re-creation process, the orthodox surgical chemotherapy or radiation process or a combination of both. Going back to the energy equation, anything which removes the obstruction to function and puts more available life energy into the body's energy bank is going to improve the chances of regaining health and, above all, the quality of lifestyle and level of well-being of the person involved.

To improve any situation in relation to the body's health and well-being, there are a number of essential parts of the process:
• The individual needs to accept responsibility for taking on the role of self-help creator and body well-being maintenance
• The mental and emotional effect of the concentration on the re-creation

of health, rather than the treatment of cancer, has an enormous effect in enabling the body to restore its normal function and to help itself to deal with the metabolic immune system and chemical abnormalities which are present at the time

• The most important thing in choosing the path to follow is to exercise the individual right to have a choice – to exercise this choice based on knowledge gained, and to follow this with enthusiasm, positivity and belief

The only true source of re-creation and maintenance of health is within each individual; all that is needed is the opportunity to be allowed to act in harmony and in accord with nature. The following chapters will deal in detail with the process of self-empowerment and the areas of obstruction to energy availability, and how to manage them.

Chapter 5
Nutrition

Hippocrates, considered the Father of Medicine, once said, 'Let your food be your medicine and your medicine be your food.' In his day, and for many centuries after, this approach to the creation and maintenance of health was possible. Unfortunately, it all went wrong in the mid-twentieth century.

Quality food and the difficulties in obtaining it

The basis of quality food is quality soil and agriculture, because the plant is totally dependent on its environment for its ability to absorb and present the nutrients that man needs to maintain physical and structural health. The origin of nutrition is always plant life: even if we live on meat, the animal which supplied the meat lived on plants (or on another animal which lived on plants). The process of health begins and ends in the soil. In a natural environment, a healthy soil, rich in minerals, watered by pure water and covered with natural healthy seed will produce plants of all types which contain the organic vitamins and minerals essential for man and other animals to maintain their existence.

Unfortunately, if you're trying to create and maintain health, you face a lot of problems in obtaining good food that will meet the body's nutritional needs with a balance of vitamins and minerals.

Minerals

In the natural course of events, the ground is rich in the required minerals.

The plants absorb these inorganic minerals and, through a chemical process, change them to organic minerals. Organic minerals are designed to let the body digest, absorb and use them effectively without creating high levels of waste matter for the body to process during this chemical exchange. Natural organic vitamins and minerals are the product of the plant chemistry and are always highly bio-available – that is, they are able to be absorbed by the body; they are released steadily throughout the digestion process.

Later in this chapter, I will discuss absorption and bio-availability in the section under supplementation, but it is important to understand that in nature all the vitamins and minerals are molecularly complete: that is, they have do not need to bond with other chemical substances to return them to a balanced state during their process through the intestines. Where molecular structures are incomplete – that is, not as they would be found in nature – and perhaps taken in too high a dose, other chemicals will be used to balance this and will be carried out of the body during the process of elimination. For example, if you take too much vitamin C, the body will use zinc to help process and control its usage of vitamin C, and zinc will be carried out of the body. Therefore you are actually taking away from the body the substance that is necessary for vitamin C usage and taking too much chemically isolated vitamin C will actually create an increase in vitamin C deficiency.

Changing soil structure

The ever-increasing use of nitrates and fertilisers has in many ways destroyed the structure of the soil, which has been further affected by heavy cropping, non-rotational farming and removal of hedgerows and trees. All these things have resulted in changes in the quality of soil. For a start, the topsoil erodes more rapidly, due to the lack of protection from natural wind breaks and the nature of its artificially treated surface structure. In many places throughout the world, dustbowls and soil erosion are major problems, and the *Earth Summit Report* of 1992 concluded that over the past 100 years, soil had been depleted of minerals by over 75 per cent in Europe and over 80 per cent in the United States of America.

Only three of the necessary 60 minerals tend to be put back into the soil in intensive agricultural practices: nitrogen, phosphorus and potassium, which are the only minerals plants require for growth. Although these produce good quantities of crops, the food is actually nutrient-deficient.

Where there are heavy quantities of nitrates in the soil, the natural minerals present are bound into the soil; even if there is an adequate availability of a mineral, such as selenium, the plant cannot access it because of the excessive nitrates in the chemical structure of the soil itself. Selenium is one of the critical minerals in the function of the immune system and is now significantly absent in most foodstuffs grown in the world today. Lincolnshire was a fine example of an area with selenium-rich soil; the carrot is a good sponge for particular minerals and Lincolnshire carrots in particular were once noted for their selenium content. However, as a result of the soil treatment over the last few decades, Lincolnshire carrots contain no selenium and are not likely to in the foreseeable future, unless the soil is renatured and the defects of chemical fertilisation finally replaced.

To indicate how the changes in the soil have occurred, tables 1 and 2 below show the change in the nutritional contents of a key number of food stuffs, as measured by McCance and Widdowson in 1936 and in a remeasurement in 1987. The figures speak for themselves. McCance and Widdowson is the official Government textbook of food contents; if you want to read further on the subject, the book is available from HM Stationery Office. On average, the mineral content of food has dropped by 45 per cent over those 50 years.

Depressingly, despite the publication of this textbook, nothing has been done at the Government level to restore the relative food values to those of sixty-odd years ago.

Table 1: Mineral content of vegetables in 1936 compared with 1987

Iron	Calcium	Magnesium
Raw carrots – 88% more	Raw carrots – 92% more	Raw carrots – 300% more
Cauliflower – 23% more	Cauliflower – 35% more	–
Old potatoes – 85% more	Old potatoes – 55% more	Old potatoes – 43% more
–	Celery – 27% more	Celery – 90% more

Table 2: Mineral content of meat/poultry/fish in 1936 compared with 1987

Iron	Calcium	Magnesium
Cod – 150% more	Cod – 210% more	–
Pork – 167% more	–	–
Chicken – 75% more	–	Chicken – 6% more
Beef – 68% more	–	–
Lamb – 38% more	Lamb – 125% more	Lamb – 15% more

Water in the plant cycle

Water is an important part of plant development, because of course it has an effect in all parts of the growth cycle. Water evaporates from the surface of the earth; at this point it is pure H_2O and carries no contaminants at all. The water rises into the sky and is processed by wind and terrain until it precipitates and falls as rain.

In the ideal situation, where the air is not polluted and the atmosphere is balanced, the water falls back to earth, on the leaves and outer surfaces of plants as well as the soil itself. It falls as snow in colder areas and waits until the appropriate time of year to thaw and flow out once more onto the land. The water filters through the different structures upon which it has landed or flowed and sinks through to underground water reservoirs, from whence pressure eventually brings it to the surface and the process of evaporation begins once more.

As the water travels down through the earth, it absorbs minerals and salts from soil and rock; thus, when it reappears as a spring, it is more enriched than when it fell as rain. This mineral-enriched water is sucked up by the roots of plants and transfers its inorganic minerals to it, along with those of the soil – which can of course be very different if the water travels considerable distances. This gives the plant the broad base of minerals which are so necessary for the process of life to continue.

We can thus see what a damaging effect the quality of the atmosphere and events which produce such things as acid rain have on the balance of nature's nutritional circle, and how important it is to correct these imbalances in the environment.

Animal foods

Animals eat the plants and drink the water which is available; where nature has not been interfered with, these animals grow healthy vibrant tissues which make them healthy and resistant to disease. Where the flesh of other animals is eaten, as long as the animal itself was healthy, then the chain of health maintenance is not broken.

Sadly, it is now exceedingly difficult to find animals, birds or even fish which are healthy, as the way that animals and bird are reared and the pollution of the seas affecting fish mean that their nutritional value is decreased. There are often also harmful side-effects from the use of hormonal additives to animal feed, hormonal interference with the development of poultry, and of course the practice of animals being fed to other animals, which resulted in the recent devastating BSE scare.

The use of antibiotics in animal development is quite commonplace and, while safety regulations have been introduced, these are only safe if they are adhered to with extreme diligence.

Artificial fertiliser versus the organic approach

In the environment when one type of food intake is used by another organism in the food chain, the leftovers are always reprocessed and sent back to the earth. Man, however, has once again failed to understand this essential piece of nature's maintenance of balance. Prior to artificial fertilisers, pesticides and growth enhancers, the compost heap was a part of every gardener's rotational process with the remains, which were returned, helping to give back to the soil that which had been taken away.

Farmers at the turn of the century used the manure from their animals, who were all naturally fed, as a means of refertilising their fields, and coupled this with careful husbandry and crop rotation to provide the variations so important for maintenance of the balance of the soil as a whole. Animal manure today may sadly contain hormone and antibiotic residue, which has significance in relation to the immune system.

There is a huge move now – happily as a result of the demand-creating supply – for all the major supermarkets and food stores to invest in organically grown foods; the amount of products and the range available is increasing all the time. This is a major improvement and is a great step forward to an awakening of the damage done to nature's production of food industry.

Why organic is better for you

When you're eating to re-create and maintain health, it's important that the food you eat is as good as possible. The vitamin and mineral content of organic food is higher than that of non-organic food. Kirlian photography – a technique that shows energy fields – show that there is a huge difference in the amount of energy available in organic and non-organic food. This is one of the reasons why it's important to eat organic food if you have cancer: because organic food puts more of the balanced life energy into the body. Organic food is produced without artificial fertilisers, herbicides or pesticides, and therefore there are no potentially harmful residues, and there is naturally balanced vitamin and mineral content. The importance of organic food as part of a health maintenance diet cannot be overemphasised.

Eating in season

It's also a good idea to follow the old precept of eating whatever food is in season. Nature knows when we need the foods we eat, and out-of-season and exotic foods are artificially ripened, which reduces their nutritional value. Eating food grown locally is also helpful, particularly when you're trying to pay back an overdraft to your energy bank; food grown locally is likely to be fresher than that shipped across the country or even a continent, because it hasn't had so far to travel and therefore arrives at the supermarket or shop more quickly after it's harvested. This gives much less time for oxidisation and life energy loss. Oxidisation is the process of decomposition; some foods go bad more quickly than others and it makes sense to eat food soon after you buy it rather than trying to store it for a long time. If you do need to store it, always unwrap it; if you keep it in the fridge, it shouldn't need extra wrapping, or use brown paper bags if you store the food out of the fridge.

Energy and elimination

As energy in the bank account increases, there is sufficient energy available to pay long overdue direct debits in the body's elimination, healing and repair cycles. This increase in elimination is a fundamental part of the body's cleansing process – to remove stored-up toxic waste from the tissues and to stimulate the mechanism of removing these from the body and eliminating them from the bloodstream, kidneys and skin.

As the process progresses, your liver can become involved in the cleansing process. This may lead to nausea and headaches, but it's important to remember that this is a positive response rather than a negative one. Your body is spending its extra energy wisely and is cleaning its home before starting a rebuilding programme – a bit like rubbing the woodwork down before you repaint it.

The balance of foodstuffs

I believe that the individual's choice of food is important, which is why I advocate a framework of foods from which you can choose rather than a strict diet which you are more likely to feel is forced on you and are therefore less likely to stick to. A softer approach means that you can pick the foods you're comfortable eating; there's little point in eating something you don't like. Listen to your body and it will tell you what it needs. As you get healthier, you'll intuitively choose the right foods and healthier options.

It's important to eat three balanced meals a day, so that the digestion and assimilation processes have time to work properly and finish. If you 'graze' all day, you use your digestion cycle all the time, acids and enzymes are released continually by your digestive system, and the body doesn't have a chance to rest. I would only recommend frequent small meals in cases where people can't physically manage sensible-sized meals.

By balanced, I mean that you need good-quality protein plus vitamins, minerals, fibre, oils and fats – including non-saturated fat, omega-3 and omega-6 fatty acids. It's important to have a choice; if you need to eat something occasionally, such as chocolate, that's fine. Vegetables and fruit will provide vitamins, minerals and fibre. Pasta, rice and grain are important forms of carbohydrate; choose organic, wholemeal varieties rather than the processed type which are refined and produce a high residue of waste when the body breaks them down.

For proteins, you can eat soya, beans, pulses, grains, cereals, nuts, meat, fish, flow, game and dairy produce. There's a protein mania in this country and people tend to think that they need more protein than they really do. Red meat in particular has a high acid residue, which upsets the body's acid-alkali balance. The excess protein is then killed off and the body has an increased need for protein; eating more red meat leads to a greater imbalance in the body and this quickly becomes a vicious circle, so try to use less acid forms of protein.

Keep dairy produce to an absolute minimum; soya milk, goat's milk and ewe's milk are good alternatives. Remember that pasteurisation is a treatment process which will remove some of the benefits of organic food, so choose unpasteurised goat's or ewe's milk; although the words organic and skimmed milk seem to be at odds, organic skimmed milk is actually one of the least harmful products. If you wish to eat eggs, keep them to a maximum of three a week, and always choose organic eggs. Although eggs have a degree of cholesterol, they also contain its antidote to balance it out.

Remember that whether you choose to be a vegan (eating no produce connected with animals), a vegetarian (eating no meat, fowl or fish) or you decide to eat meat, as long as your diet is balanced you can be fit. It's when your diet isn't balanced that you're likely to have problems, and remember that it's harder for vegans to eat a balanced diet because of the dietary restrictions.

Use foods that are easy to digest, to give the maximum input into the energy bank account but make sure the body uses the least possible energy when assimilating the food. Avoid highly processed or refined foods, additives and stimulants such as tea and coffee, which act as credit cards in the energy bank.

Appendix 2 shows the recommended daily amount of vitamins and minerals required by the average adult, plus what I recommend for people who have cancer, together with what the vitamins and minerals do in the body.

Starting to re-create health

When starting the programme to re-create health, use the following diet (on alternate days) for the first two weeks, in addition to a daily supplement of food state vitamins and minerals. Then follow either the chemotherapy or the general diet, as appropriate.

The food should always be of organic origin, preferably locally grown or sourced from a known compost-producing outlet, and it is best for the food to be unwrapped and obtained as soon as possible after harvest, so it's at its freshest and uncontaminated by any chemical residues on the packaging.

First two weeks

For drinks between meals, use black dandelion coffee, no-caff (coffee substitute made from figs and chiccory, available from health stores), grape juice, apple juice or fruit tea, plus at least 2 litres/3 ½ pints of the purest water available (see pages 112 for methods of producing this in the home). If you have a juicer, organic cabbage and carrot juice are beneficial; they may be mixed with apple to improve palatability. Don't drink with meals, as this dilutes your digestive enzymes and also extends your stomach.

Day 1:

Breakfast – whole oats soaked overnight in apple juice, with grated raw apple and soaked or simmered raisins

Mid-morning – slippery elm drink and seedless grapes

Lunch – varied raw salad with grated carrot, beetroot and watercress together with nut or soya savoury and one or two rye crispbread. Melon or grapes to follow

Mid-afternoon – slippery elm drink and seedless grapes

Evening meal – any vegetarian savoury that does not include dairy produce, together with broccoli, carrots and one other green vegetable. Apple or grapes to follow

On retiring – one cup of slippery elm drink

Day 2:

Breakfast – one slice of wholemeal toast with vegetarian margarine and grilled or baked tomatoes. Half a grapefruit

Mid-morning – slippery elm drink and seedless grapes

Lunch – varied raw salad with grated carrot, beetroot and watercress with nut or soya savoury and one or two rye crispbread. Melon or grapes to follow

Mid-afternoon – slippery elm drink and seedless grapes

Evening meal – steamed or grilled white fish with broccoli and one or two other vegetables of your choice (excluding potatoes). Half a grapefruit

On retiring – one cup of slippery elm drink

Repeat days one and two in rotation

Chemotherapy diet

Follow this diet for the day before chemotherapy, during treatment, and one day after. Drink between one and a half and two litres of mineral water daily, plus vitamin supplements as recommended.

Morning – hot water (still mineral water from a glass bottle) with a slice of lemon, if desired

Breakfast – slippery elm drink with stewed apple and soaked or simmered raisins, if desired

Mid-morning – slippery elm drink

Lunch – carrots, parsnips, turnips and swede mashed with a little vegetarian margarine

Mid-afternoon – slippery elm drink

Evening meal – mashed vegetables (as per lunchtime)

On retiring – one cup of slippery elm drink

General diet

Follow this diet after the two-week starter diet. You need to omit all dairy produce from your diet; use soya milk (such as Provamel without added calcium) or organic oat milk instead. Don't drink with meals. Drink at least 2 litres/3 ½ pints of the purest water available (preferably taken at blood heat/approx 36°C/ 98°F) during the day; do not add fruit juice or herbal teas, as the water should act as part of the flushing mechanism of the body. If you wish to drink other drinks between meals, use chamomile, ginger or mint herbal tea, no-caff or dandelion coffee. You should also take a vitamin supplement as directed.

On rising – glass of organic apple juice half diluted with warm water

Breakfast – choice of:

• Organic whole oats soaked overnight in organic oat milk or organic apple juice with grated raw apple

• Organic whole oats made into porridge with soya milk or oat milk; fresh apple

• One or two piece of rye toast with pure spread and grated raw carrot

• Selection of fresh fruit – apple, melon or grapefruit

Lunch – large varied raw salad from organic produce; vary both the content and colour of the food, including items such as:

• Lettuce

• White cabbage

• Radishes

• Onions

• Cucumber

• Chiccory

• Grated carrot

• Raw beetroot (grated or cooked unvinegared organic beetroot – hot or cold)

   Plus a selection from:

• Milled nuts

• Soya protein

• Beans or pulses

• Tinned or fresh salmon or tuna (occasionally)

   Plus: one or two rye crispbread with organic or vegan spread, if desired; or a small organic baked jacket potato up to three times a week

   Plus: half a grapefruit or some grapes, if desired

Evening meal – one of the following proteins:

- Vegetarian protein (excluding dairy produce) at least three times a week
- Grilled or steamed white fish or salmon
- Free range poultry
- Organic red meat (no more than once a week)

Plus: seasonal vegetables – particularly broccoli and root vegetables (other than potatoes), with cabbage or spinach. The vegetables should be steamed, not overheated, and should be cooked fresh for each meal

Plus: apple, pear, grapefruit or grapes if desired.

Cooked vegetables can always be replaced by raw or salad vegetables.

Detoxification

Detoxification is part of the body's healing mechanism, during which you can suffer from headaches, nausea and tiredness for a short period. Do not take anything to combat this; let your body complete its cycle and you'll feel better.

Food preparation

All organic food should be washed thoroughly before use; although no chemicals have been used in producing it, the food will have been affected by rainwater, which contains a cocktail of unpleasant chemicals.

If you use inorganic food, you need to remove the outer layers, particularly in the case of fruit, because pesticides lodge in the skin. As the skin contains the biggest concentration of vitamins and minerals, you're actually throwing away the best bit – so you're better off using organic food. There's little excuse nowadays for not using organic food, as it's very widely available in supermarkets and is not expensive. And you'll actually find that you need to eat less of it to get the quantity of vitamins and minerals your body needs;

we overeat simply because our body is undernourished. If we eat food which has better nutritional values, we need less and our body becomes more efficient at elimination, which helps to fill our energy bank.

Raw

By and large, raw vegetables and fruit are best because the energy in them isn't affected by cooking, so there is no interference with the natural balances and contents. Carrots are the one exception as the bio-availability is increased by gentle cooking, but this is more than offset by the energy lost by heating them.

Steaming

Steaming is the best method of cooking vegetables and fish, because the vitamins and minerals are not boiled away in the cooking water. Also, there is a shorter cooking time and less exposure to heat, which means that the life energy of the food is less diminished then it is by other cooking methods.

Grilling

Grilling is good for fish and meat because no fat needs to be added and no fat is absorbed, unlike with frying.

Stir-frying

Stir-frying in a little extra virgin olive oil (or just water) is good for vegetables because the cooking time is very short and the vegetables therefore retain their crispness and nutritional value.

Microwaving

Evidence shows that mobile phones may be dangerous; similar vibrations are used in microwave cooking. It's an intense process where the food cooks from the centre outwards, so there is a high level of destruction in the contents. Although there is no hard scientific evidence, I feel that microwaving is a form of cooking best avoided as it interferes with the energy of the food.

Other methods

There is a lot of evidence to suggest that blackened foods have a higher carcinogenic content. Gas barbecues – which use lava coals rather than charcoal – are better, but it's best to use this as only an occasional method of cooking. If you already have cancer, avoid it completely. Baking is fine but lengthy exposure to heat wrecks the nutritional value. Try to use the shortest possible cooking time. With boiling, a lot of nutrients are lost in the water, which is then thrown away; steaming, as mentioned above, is better, particularly as you can use the water as stock for soups.

The healthy approach to eating

It is important when you eat to concentrate on the food rather than try to do several things at once. If you eat in a relaxed fashion and appreciate the quality of the food you're eating and enjoy what it's giving to you, your body will have a chance to digest the food properly. Positive input creates a positive response. If you eat in front of the TV or while reading or while rushing around trying to snatch bites between tasks, you won't be able to concentrate on the food and it won't do its job properly.

Supplementation

Chemical isolates versus food state minerals

Supplements today are made from chemical isolates, which are the only legal source of minerals and vitamins; they may be produced chemically or taken from plants, and are packed in excipients – that is, the balance of the tablets which are not active ingredients. Isolated chemical vitamins and minerals differ in excipient quality, the amount of active ingredients and production processes, but none of them are presented as they are in natural food.

My father had been a naturopath for thirty years, and he taught me that the food itself was the important thing and supplements tended to treat the symptoms of a disease rather than the cause. However, as we have already seen, food has become so devalued that it's unable to do its job properly and the body needs supplements. After ten years I grudgingly began to use supplements, but I was not happy until twelve years ago when I was introduced to *food state* vitamins and minerals.

Food state vitamins and minerals – which are produced in the US – are renatured; that is, they are 'grown back' into the food matrix. With a traditional supplement, the chemical isolate of the inorganic mineral is simply added to ingredients to bind them and bulk out the tablet; the finished product is never found in this form in natural food. However, with food state minerals, the chemical isolate of the inorganic mineral is put into a tank that contains a nutrient-rich broth. The mineral is taken up by the yeast in the broth and grown for 24–48 hours; then the cells walls of the yeast are broken down and removed. This leaves the food state nutrient with a complete food-based delivery system; it's spray-dried, added to ingredients to bind them and bulk out the tablet, and the finished product is exactly the same as is found in natural foods. This means in a total food matrix, all the necessary minerals can be dealt with in this fashion.

The same is true of vitamins. If we take our old friend vitamin C: in traditional supplements, the synthesised vitamin (ascorbic acid) is added to ingredients to bind them and bulk out the tablet; the finished product isn't found in natural food. With the food state vitamin supplement, the vitamin is added to a tank containing the appropriate food matrix (in the case of vitamin C, this is a citrus pulp concentrate), left to react for 8-16 hours, and this leaves the food state nutrient with a complete food-based delivery system. As with the minerals, it's spray-dried, added to ingredients to bind them and bulk out the tablet, and the finished product is once again as is found in natural foods.

Why is this so important? Let's consider how the body uses food. The food matrix delivers nutrients to a specific area of the gut. If we think of the gut as a supermarket with its shelves stocked by a balanced diet, the body is able to *go shopping* for the vitamins and minerals it requires that day. The body's needs change on a day-to-day basis; you eat during the day to give the body the choice of what it needs, and it decides what to use. For example, it may take all the vitamin C on the shelves on one day, and none at all on the next. With a balanced diet, the body knows the layout of the supermarket and everything is unwrapped, so the body can see exactly what it needs and take it. Food state minerals and vitamins behave in exactly the same way as foods and the body is able to recognise them.

However, with traditional supplements that are chemical isolates only, the body has more difficulty going shopping. The layout of the body's super-market has changed and isn't signposted in the way that the food matrix signposted its shelves. All the packages are wrapped, so the body has to unwrap each one before it can see if the mineral or vitamin is the one it wants. All this uses extra energy and means there's more rubbish to get rid of, so it's clear that food state minerals and vitamins are more efficient.

Appendix 3 shows the approximate correlation between food state nutrients and traditional supplements.

Water

Water is hugely important to our diet. Our bodies are made up of between 75 and 85 per cent water, so it's critical that we drink enough. Dehydration is a very common cause of illness; if you wait until you're thirsty, it's too late. You need to drink between three and a half and four pints of water a day; if it's hot or you're taking exercise, you'll need to increase the quantity of water you drink accordingly.

Tap water

The quality of tap water is not good; apart from the chemicals used to treat the water – such as chlorine and fluoride – to make it safe for human consumption, the water often travels through old piping and may end up containing a great deal of lead or asbestos, and some areas of the country have a lot of nitrates in their water table because of intensive use of artificial fertiliser in agriculture. Tap water has between 50 and 900 parts per million of dissolved impurities.

Bottled water

Surprisingly, bottled mineral water is not as good for you as the marketing gurus would have us believe. There are two forms of minerals: organic and inorganic. Inorganic minerals are non-vegetable and non-animal, and the body can't use them effectively. Most brands of mineral and spring water contain a lot of inorganic minerals, as a result of the agricultural process destroying the soil through which the water is filtered. These inorganic minerals can leave a residue in our bodies and can cause a wide range of problems and illnesses, including arthritis, varicose veins, emphysema, kidney stones and constipation.

Excessive mineral content can also damage our health. Spring or mineral water has up to 2600 parts per million of dissolved impurities.

If you use bottled water, it's better to use water from glass bottles – because unless a plastic bottle is made from very high quality plastic, its chemical constituents leak into the water and contribute to the production of cancer-forming free radicals in the body.

Still water is better for you than carbonated water. Your body spends the whole day breathing out carbon dioxide, so why make your body work harder by giving it extra quantities to remove? Remember that your body can't absorb oxygen as efficiently when carbon dioxide takes up the space.

Filtered water

Filtering water can help improve the taste and remove the impurities present in tap water. The filtration process is the removal of physical particles and dissolved substances – such as chlorine and pesticides – by physical means. Barrier filters made of compressed cellulose, spun rayon fibre or processed ceramic can remove mud, clay, sand, silt and scal, making the water much clearer. Carbon blocks and granules filter out dissolved gases and other organic substances.

However, there are limits to the amount of material that can be removed from the water. The effectiveness of the system depends on the quality of the filter; you will also need to change the filter regularly as there will be a build-up of residues in the filter. There's always the chance that the filter may become clogged and contaminate the water with material contained in the filters; this is particularly true of bacteria.

If using the filtration method, I advise that you filter the water twice before using it, and change the filter in the jug more frequently than the manufacturers advise, to make sure that it's working most efficiently.

Distilled water

Distillation is where the water is heated to 100°C and the steam is condensed. Distilled water is the main means of purifying water in laboratories;

however, it can't be used for water that contains high levels of dissolved solids, such as sea water or bore water. The boiling process removes oxygen so the water tastes harsh, and the water may also contain dead bacteria (endotoxins) which act as food for live bacteria. Distillers also suffer from scale formation and are therefore high-maintenance.

Reverse osmosis

Osmosis is a natural function; if a semi-permeable membrane is placed between dirty and clean water, the clean water naturally migrates through the membrane to the dirty water. Reverse osmosis where the dirty water is purified under pressure by being forced through the semi-permeable membrane to join the clean water. There is a self-cleaning mechanism involved, because the reject water 'backwashes' the membrane and carries away bacteria and other pollutants. Because the movement of the water through the membrane depends on the chemical bonding of the molecules rather than the physical size of the molecules, the membrane does not act in the same way as a filter, but it is effective against most pollutants and removes a significant amount of bacteria.

However, the process is very wasteful as between 50 and 80 per cent of the water is rejected; this can cause problems in disposing of the waste water. The membrane will also need to be replaced regularly, and there is a risk of the dirty water being let through the rings that hold the membrane in place. The process doesn't kill the bacteria, so any that are not taken out by the process will still be alive in the clean water.

Cold vaporisation

Cold vaporisation was developed by Dr Davoid Tajer to replicate a process that occurs in nature, where the suns warms the sea and land water and vapour rises into the atmosphere. As the vapour rises, impurities – including toxic waste – come out of the vapour; then when the vapour reaches a certain height it chills and condenses back to water – which turns into rain.

With cold vaporisation, the water is evaporated at between 18°C and 34°C in a vacuum chamber. The water vapour is too thin to support the weight of the molecules of any dissolved gases or inorganic material, so the system removes metals, bacteria, suspended solids and chemicals.

The vapour is then taken up into a cooling system, and moves through a vortex into a collecting tank; this creates movement and energy in the water. It's then circulated into a second vortex, and the result is pure, energised H_2O.

Supplementation and the concept of eating to get well

The whole basis of self-empowerment in relation to chemical energy is to understand that the body must be offered the full spectrum of nutritional requirements in a form that it can recognise on a daily basis. As I mentioned previously, food no longer provides this without some form of supplementation.

Over the last two years I have been using a particular form of supplementation which has helped many people to produce quite staggering results in the maintenance and development of health. In November 1998 I was introduced to this concept of the mixture of food state vitamins and minerals, a pre and pro-biotic and a pure water enhanced with the energy of tissue salts. From that point on I rapidly converted the whole of my approach to supplementation to embrace this concept completely.

As already explained, the food state vitamins and minerals offer to the body vitamins and minerals in a readily recognisable form, with a delivery mechanism to make sure that they reach the right place and can be fully used and all of the excess and waste product readily and easily removed. The formula uses a multivitamin/multimineral tablet which contains all the necessary vitamins and minerals in this food state presentation.

Coupled to this is a Fos-a-dophilus, which is a pre and pro-biotic of very high quality, which is necessary to allow the intestine to function effectively so as to absorb the nutritional intake presented to it. Pro-biotics are very well-known nowadays and they are of course a process of delivering the highly necessary beneficial bacteria to the correct part of the intestine, allowing these to grow and function normally – a very large percentage at present is destroyed by the nutritional process that we have developed. The pre-biotic part of the capsule is less well known. The Fos is a carbohydrate chain which protects the acidophilus portion of the process (the pro-biotic) and enables it to be delivered with little interference to the right part of the intestinal tract. It then provides food for the bacteria to develop and at the same time suppresses the activity of the negative bacteria, which need to be dealt with to promote effective absorption and function.

To these two elements the formula has added a water purified by a cold vaporisation process, energised by the use of vortices, and is enhanced with the energy of tissue salts. The latter works with the basic cell resonance and, by helping to create this balance, enables all the other parts of the formula to work far more effectively; it acts like a turbocharger on an engine. This in turn provides a nutritional response which enables all other food and nutritional matter consumed to be dealt with more effectively and dramatically increases the amount of energy as a result of the process.

This formula works with the energy at the subtle levels as well as the chemical level and has been outstandingly successful with thousands of people who have already been using this formula.

When giving advice to people on the creation and maintenance of health – and indeed optimal health – particularly when cancer is involved in the equation, I have used the dietary approach as outlined earlier, but always supported it with this formula, which combines food state vitamins and minerals but also uses fructo-oligosaccharides and a slightly different balance of contents. This has helped people to cope with the rigours of chemotherapy or radiotherapy or even a combination of both, with much reduced discomforts and side-effects. The basic formula is an ongoing part of life, because it seeks to replace what is missing in food; as long as we eat the food that we produce at present, then we should take this support formula to give us the basic nutrition to enable us to maintain optimum health (see Rappha, on page 215).

Eating for life

The whole process of eating to maintain health and well-being is something which can be done by each of us individually, and is something for which we have to take a personal responsibility. The dietary advice offers choices in as many areas as possible and the formula discussed above liberates the energy within the body, which helps our intuition guide us into making the right choices at the right time. To get the right combination of formula – the strengths vary – I have been using a hair energy test which establishes compatability within this process and highlights if there are any areas where an extra intake of one specific vitamin or mineral is needed.

I have found many people astounded by how easy the whole process of eating for life really is, and of course the great fact to be realised is that any treatment is being supported and its side effects confirmed, but the whole process is that of prevention of disease. We all have cancer cells within us all the time, but in a healthy body the immune system keeps these in balance. By creating a healthy body we maintain a healthy immune system and, as nature intended, the body enjoys health and well-being.

It is important not to see yourself as going on a diet but rather see each meal as it truly is, nature's gift of all the nutritional elements needed for the creation and maintenance of chemical energy. There is an old saying that you are what you eat, and this is as true now as it was thousands of years ago.

Soups & Starters

Lentil, Tomato & Barley Soup

100g/4oz/$^2/_3$ cup brown or green lentils
50g/2oz/$^1/_3$ cup pot barley
1 large red onion, finely sliced
2 sticks celery, finely diced
2 cloves garlic, finely chopped
2 carrots, scrubbed and finely diced
1 400g/12-oz tin tomatoes
1.2 litres/2 pints/5 cups vegetable stock
1 teaspoon fresh basil, finely shredded
1 tablespoon miso
Salt & freshly ground black pepper

Put the lentils and barley into a deep saucepan and cover with boiling water
Leave to soak overnight, drain and wash through with cold water.

Rinse out the pan and add all the ingredients except the basil and miso. Put
on a high heat and bring to the boil. Cover and simmer for 30 minutes until
both lentils and barley are tender. Add the basil. Remove a little of the
liquor and mix it with the miso to make a paste; pour this back into the soup
and stir in. Season as necessary and serve piping hot.

RECIPES ON THIS AND THE FOLLOWING PAGES ALL SERVE 4 PEOPLE

Potage Bonne Femme

2 tablespoons olive oil
1 medium onion, roughly chopped
750g/1½lb potatoes, scrubbed and roughly chopped
500g/1lb carrots, scraped and roughly chopped
1.2 litres/2 pints/5 cups vegetable stock
Salt & freshly ground black pepper
4 tablespoons parsley, chopped

Heat the oil in a large, heavy saucepan. Add the onion and cook until soft, over a medium heat. Add the potatoes and carrots and toss well to coat in the oil. Add the stock, salt and pepper and turn the heat up to high. Bring to the boil, cover and simmer until all the vegetables are tender.

Pour into a liquidizer or pass through a mouli. Return the soup to the pan, reheat and season to taste. Pour into individual bowls and sprinkle with the chopped parsley.

Cold Tomato & Avacado Soup

4 medium tomatoes, peeled, deseeded and chopped
1 large onion, finely chopped
1 sweet red pepper, deseeded and finely chopped
2 large avocados, peeled and chopped
1.2 litres/2 pints/5 cups tomato juice
1 tablespoon lemon juice
1 tablespoon fresh basil leaves, finely shredded
Salt & freshly ground black pepper
2 tablespoons parsley, chopped

Put all the ingredients into a blender, bar the seasoning, and blitz. When smooth, season and chill for at least two hours. Pour into bowls and sprinkle with parsley.

Jerusalem Artichoke Soup

2 tablespoons olive oil
1 large red onion, finely sliced
750g/1$\frac{1}{2}$lb Jerusalem artichokes, scrubbed, trimmed and roughly chopped
I strip orange peel
1.2 litres/2 pints/5 cups vegetable stock
Salt & freshly ground black pepper
2 tablespoons parsley

Heat the oil in a heavy bottomed saucepan and stir in the onion over medium heat. Cook until translucent. Add the artichokes, orange and stock, and bring to the boil. Cover and simmer until the artichokes are cooked through. Purée the soup, return to the pan and season. Serve garnished with a little parsley

Chestnut & Brussels Sprout Soup

A good, warming soup for winter, the flavour of the chestnuts comes through loud and clear. You can used tinned whole chestnuts if the idea of skinning them yourself is just too much.

100g/4oz chestnuts
25g/1oz olive oil or margarine
1 red onion, finely sliced
200g/7oz potatoes, peeled and diced large
750g/1½lb Brussels sprouts, cut into quarters
600ml/1 pint/2½ cups vegetable stock
a pinch of grated nutmeg
150ml/¼pint/⅔ cup milk
4 tablespoons cream
salt & freshly ground black pepper
2 tablespoons chives, to garnish

Make slits in the chestnuts and roast them on a baking sheet in an oven preheated to 200°C/400°F/gas 6 for 15-20 minutes. Leave to cool and peel Make them into a crumble.

Melt the butter in a heavy based pan and sauté the onion until softened but not browned. Add the potatoes and Brussels sprouts and coat well with the butter. Pour over the stock and bring to the boil; then cover and simmer very gently for 10 minutes. When the vegetables are soft, remove from the heat and cool a little before puréeing in a liquidiser.

Return to the pan and stir in the nutmeg, milk, cream and seasoning. Garnish with the chives and serve steaming.

Caponata

According to Mary Taylor Simeti, in her wonderful *Sicilian Food*, caponata 'is thought to have originated as seagoing fare, since it keeps well because of the vinegar'.

2-3 aubergines, cut into 2.5-cm/1-in cubes

salt

4 ripe fresh tomatoes, peeled, deseeded & chopped

125ml/4fl oz/$\frac{1}{2}$ cup extra-virgin olive oil

1 medium onion, finely chopped

6 stalks celery, cut into 2.5-cm/1-in lengths

200g/7oz green olives, pitted

4-5 tablespoons capers

50g/2oz/$\frac{1}{3}$ cup raisins

50g/2oz/$\frac{2}{3}$ cup pinenuts

2 tablespoons vinegar

2 tablespoons sugar

salt & freshly ground black pepper

Put the aubergine cubs into a colander, cover liberally with salt and leave to drain for about an hour. Rinse and dry. Meantime, cook the tomatoes in a small pan with 1 tablespoon of the olive oil and a little salt for 5 minutes until soft and then mash with a fork and set aside.

Heat 6 tablespoons of the oil in a large, heavy-based frying pan and add the aubergine. Fry until soft, drain on kitchen roll and set aside in a bowl. Add the rest of the oil and sauté the onion, celery, olives, capers, raisins and pinenuts until the celery and onion are softened. Stir in the vinegar and cook until it evaporates. Then sprinkle over the sugar and add the aubergines. Stir thoroughly and season to taste. Serve warm or cold.

Baked Rice & Peas

Use brown rice in this dish; it is one of the most easily digested grains.
Shelling peas can be remarkably theraputic; equally you may think it the most
boring job in the world, but it is well worth the effort in this dish. This
is comfort food!

200g/7oz/1¼ cups brown rice
200g/7oz/1¼cups green peas, shelled weight
4 tablespoons olive oil
50g/2oz Parmesan cheese
salt & freshly ground black pepper
200g/7oz vegan cheese, grated

Preheat the oven to 190°C/375°F/gas 5.

Bring a pan of salted water to the boil and add the rice. Cook for 10-12
minutes and then add the peas; continue cooking for a couple more minutes.
When the rice is tender, drain and put into a lightly greased casserole. Drizzle over
the oil and Parmesan, and season. Add the cheese and bake in the oven for about
15 minutes, until there is a good crusty top.

Serve immediately.

RECIPES ON THIS AND THE FOLLOWING PAGES ALL SERVE 4 PEOPLE

Salads

Tricolour Pepper Salad

1 green pepper, deseeded and diced

1 red pepper, deseeded and diced

1 yellow pepper, deseeded and diced

4 sticks celery, finely sliced

1 tablespoon red onion, finely chopped

1 large clove garlic, finely sliced

6 tablespoons walnuts, chopped

6–8 tablespoons vinaigrette

Combine all the salad ingredients in a bowl, pour over the vinaigrette and season well. Chill for an hour or so and serve.

Roasted Tomato & Pasta Salad

4 large beef tomatoes, peeled and cut in half

a little olive oil for roasting

1 large aubergine, cubed

250g/$\frac{1}{2}$ lb/2 cups wholewheat fussili

3 spring onions or shallots, finely sliced

1 large green pepper, deseeded and diced

3 tablespoons black olives, stoned

2 tablespoons fresh herbs – oregano, thyme & parsley

3 tablespoons extra virgin olive oil

1 tablespoon balsamic vinegar

Salt & freshly ground black pepper

Preheat the oven to 190°C/375°F/gas 5. Put the tomatoes, cut side down, onto a baking tray, season with salt and pepper, and drizzle with the olive oil. Roast in the oven for 40 minutes or so until the sides of the tomatoes are beginning to blacken. Remove from the pan and set aside to cool.

In the same pan, over a high heat, toss the aubergine cubes until they are lightly browned all over. You may need to add more olive oil. Remove from the heat and allow to cool.

Drop the fussili into a large pan of boiling, salted water and boil hard until the pasta is cooked al dente. Drain immediately and refresh under cool water. Drizzle with a little olive oil and leave until cold. Place in a large bowl, and add the tomatoes, roughly chopped, the aubergines, spring onions, green pepper and olives and toss to mix. Sprinkle over the herbs. Make the vinaigrette by mixing the oil, vinegar and seasoning to taste in a jam jar, and pour over the salad. Toss and serve.

Middle Eastern Tomato Salad

The use of green chilli in this dish makes a refreshing change from our tomato salads.

6–8 flavourful tomatoes, peeled and cut into a large dice
juice of 1 lemon
1 green chilli, deseeded and finely minced
4 tablespoons olive oil
2 tablespoons coriander
sea salt and freshly ground black pepper

Toss all the ingredients together and serve.

Tasty Rice Salad

Pinenuts are rich in iron. Rice has been cultivated for centuries and may have originated in India, spreading to the rest of the world from there; certainly the Chinese have been known to use rice as a staple for over 5,000 years. Brown rice, being less refined than the white varieties, is richer in nutrients and gluten-free.

50g/2oz dried porcini mushrooms, tossed in a pan with a little olive oil
100g/4oz brown rice
6 artichoke hearts, cooked and quartered
6 tablespoons toasted pinenuts
3–4 tomatoes, peeled and quartered
1 small red onion, peeled and finely chopped
1 clove garlic, finely chopped
2 tablespoons lemon juice
2 tablespoons parsley
salt & freshly ground black pepper

for the dressing:
3 tablespoons extra-virgin olive oil
1 tablespoon balsamic vinegar
1 teaspoon honey
1 teaspoon moutard de Meaux
freshly ground black pepper

lettuce leaves, to serve

Put the porcini in a bowl and pour over boiling water to cover. Set aside for 30 minutes.

Meantime, combine all the ingredients in a large bowl and mix gently but thoroughly. When the mushrooms have reconstituted, squeeze the soaking liquor from them and rinse thoroughly in several changes of water to rid them of any grit. Heat a little olive oil in a pan and toss in the mushrooms. Stir until cooked and add to the salad just before dressing it. Pour over the dressing and leave overnight to marinate to allow the flavours to come through. Serve on a bed of leaves.

Middle Eastern Bread Salad

2–3 wholewheat pita breads

1 small red onion, peeled and choppped small

500g/1lb tomatoes, peeled and chopped

2 cloves garlic, crushed with a little salt

1 cucumber, chopped into a 2.5-cm/1-in dice

1 green pepper, deseeded and diced

juice of 1 lemon

2 tablespoons olive oil

2 tablespoons plain yoghurt

3 tablespoons flat-leaf parsley, finely chopped

2 tablespoons mint, finely chopped

2 tablespoons coriander, finely chopped

salt & freshly ground black pepper

Slit and open up the pita breads and toast them until crisp. Break them into small pieces and set aside. In a serving bowl put the onions, tomatoes, garlic, cucumber, pepper and lemon juice, and mix well. Season. Mix the oil and yoghurt together and stir into the vegetables, together with the herbs. Finally add the bread and toss thoroughly before serving.

Bean & Avacado Salad

500g/1lb French beans, topped and tailed

1 400-g/14-oz tin flageolet beans, drained

1 400-g/14-oz tin butter beans, drained

1 400-g/14-oz tin kidney beans, drained

2 large avocadoes, peeled, stoned and diced

2 tablespoons onion, finely chopped

1 clove garlic, finely chopped

2 tablespoons flat-leaved parsley, chopped

5 tablespoons olive oil

juice of half a lemon

sea salt & freshly ground black pepper

Cook the French beans in a large pan of boiling, salted water for 5 minutes, until slightly cooked but still crunchy. Drain, refresh under cold water and set aside to cool.

Meantime, assemble the other ingredients bar those for the vinaigrette in a large bowl and mix thoroughly. Add the French beans and season with sea salt Make the vinaigrette in a jam jar and pour over the salad. Toss well and serve. This goes well with a robust salad made of raddichio and cos lettuce.

Robust Cabbage & Raisin Salad

Honey is versatile and comes in many flavours from acacia to clover to heather; it can be used instead of sugar as a sweetener, and it makes a good substitute in vinaigrettes when you want a more robust flavour. Try to get hazelnuts from a health food store; they tend to have better quality nuts than the supermarket.

2 tablespoons hazelnuts
1 small white cabbage with a good heart, shredded
2–3 sticks celery, finely chopped
2–3 dessert apples, grated
2 tablespoons plump raisins
1 tablespoon mint leaves, chopped
1 tablespoon chives, finely snipped
3 tablespoons runny honey
3 teaspoons white wine vinegar
salt & black pepper

Toast the hazelnuts in a small pan over medium heat until they just begin to colour. Combine the nuts, vegetables, fruits and herbs in a large bowl, and make a dressing from the honey and vinegar. Season with salt and pepper and serve.

Main Courses

Lasagne

250g/8oz wholewheat lasagne

2 tablespoons olive oil

1 large onion, finely sliced

2 cloves garlic, finely crushed

2 sticks celery, finely sliced

1 can (400g/14oz) nut savoury, mashed

1 can (400g/14oz) chopped tomatoes

1 tablespoon tomato purée

for the sauce:

50g/2oz margarine

2 tablespoons cornflour

pinch dry mustard powder

600ml/1 pint/2½ cups soya milk

100g/4oz vegan cheese, grated

sea salt & freshly ground black pepper

2 tablespoons vegan cheese, grated for the topping

Preheat the oven to 200°C/400°F/gas 6. Put the lasagne sheets into a large pan of boiling, salted water and cook until tender. Drain.

Heat the oil in a large, heavy-based frying pan and toss in the onions, garlic and celery. Sauté until the onions are lightly coloured. Add the nut savoury, tomatoes and tomato purée and stir to combine thoroughly. Cook for a few minutes over a low heat.

Meanwhile make the sauce by heating the margarine in a small saucepan over medium heat and stir in the cornflour and dry mustard powder. Cook for one minute. Gradually stir in the soya milk and, when the sauce has thickened, add the cheese and seasonings.

Line the bottom of a deep, well-oiled pan with slices of lasagne. Then layer in the meat mixture and top with the cheese sauce. Repeat until all the ingredients are used up, finishing off with a layer of lasagne. Reserve 2 tablespoons of the cheese sauce for the top of the pie and sprinkle over the final 2 tablespoons of grated cheese.

Cook, uncovered, in the oven for 40 minutes until the top of the lasagne is nicely browned. Serve with a tasty green salad.

Pasta Siciliana

Redolent flavours burst through in this dish; the use of saffron gives the pasta a glowing colour compared with the bright green of the broccoli, and the currants and pinenuts give it plenty of bite.

500g/1lb bucatini
1kg/2lb broccoli, cut down to florets
2 tablespoons olive oil
1 onion, finely sliced
3 cloves garlic, finely crushed with a little salt
3 tablespoons capers
2 tablespoons currants
2 tablespoons pinenuts, lightly toasted in a dry pan for a minute or two
a few powdered saffron threads
salt & freshly ground black pepper

Put the bucatini into a large pan of boiling, salted water and cook until *al dente*.

Put the broccoli florets into a steamer and steam over plenty of boiling, salted water until just tender but still with plenty of crunch.

In a large, heavy-based frying pan heat the oil and sauté the onion and garlic until soft. Add the capers, currants, pinenuts and saffron and stir well. Then add the broccoli and season with plenty of pepper and salt to taste.

Serve in a large bowl in which you have tossed the pasta with half of the broccoli mixture and place the balance of the mixture on the top of the pasta.

Chinese Egg Noodles with Mushrooms

This recipe is taken from Oded Schwartz's *Fresh & Fast Vegetarian.*

4 tablespoons peanut oil

100g/4oz shallots, roughly chopped

2 cloves garlic, finely chopped

300g/10oz brown cap mushrooms, cleaned and sliced

200g/7oz oyster mushrooms, broken into chunks

100g/4oz fresh shitake, stems removed and sliced

4 tablespoons dark soy sauce

400ml/14fl oz vegetable stock

500g/1lb fresh or dried Chinese egg noodles

salt

2 tablespoons fresh dill to garnish

Heat the oil in a wok or heavy-based frying pan. Add the shallots and garlic and fry over a high heat until the mixture starts to brown. Add the three sorts of mushroom and continue frying until they begin to emit their juices. Add the soy sauce and fry for a minute or two, then add the stock. Bring to the boil, reduce the heat and simmer over a low heat for 10 minutes.

Prepare the noodles. If fresh, boil for 3 minutes, testing all the time – they should be tender but firm – then drain well. For dry noodles, see manufacturer's instructions.

Increase the heat under the mushrooms, add the drained noodles and cook, folding the noodles into the mushroom sauce, until almost all the liquid has evaporated and the noodles are glossy. Adjust the salt, sprinkle with the dill and serve hot, accompanied by a fresh green salad.

Perfumed Tofu

A second contribution from Oded Schwartz's *Fresh & Fast Vegetarian*, a lovely collection of original and appealing recipes.

peanut oil, for brushing
8 slices French bread, roughly 2.5cm/1in thick
1 teaspoon Chinese sesame oil, for brushing
1 onion, thinly sliced into rings
1 carrot, cleaned and cut into julienne strips
1 red pepper, deseeded and cut into julienne strips
2 fat cloves garlic, peeled and thinly sliced
500g/1lb tofu, divided into 4 portions
4 small sprigs fresh thyme
4 sticks lemongrass, 2.5cm/1in long
4 cardamom pods, broken
3 tablespoons soy sauce
2 tablespoons Chinese Sesame oil

Heat the oven to 190°C/375°F/gas 5. Brush a large baking tin with the peanut oil and arrange the bread slices in it. Sprinkle each slice with about 1 teaspoon of Chinese sesame oil. Put the tray in the bottom of the preheated oven and bake for 10–12 minutes or until the bread is browned and crisp.

Cut out 4 25-cm/10-in square pieces of kitchen foil. Brush the centre of each square generously with peanut oil. Place the onion, carrot, pepper and garlic at the centre of each square and lay the tofu on top. Top with the thyme, lemongrass and cardamom. Sprinkle with soy sauce and sesame oil. Seal the parcel by crimping the edges together. Place on a baking tray and bake in the oven for 10–12 minutes. Transfer the parcels onto individual plates, and place the bread in front. Allow diners to tear the parcels, so the delicious juices can soak the bread.

Braised Lentils & Bulgur Wheat

50g/2oz Puy lentils

7g/¼oz dried porcini mushrooms

300g/10oz shallots, peeled and left whole

bunch of organic baby carrots, trimmed and washed

2 tablespoons fresh thyme leaves

250ml/8fl oz vegetable stock

2 tablespoons olive oil

sea salt & freshly ground black pepper

for the bulgur:

500g/1lb bulgur wheat

2 onions, roughly chopped

2–3 tablespoons vegetable oil

½ teaspoon fresh marjoram leaves

sea salt & freshly ground black pepper

Cover the lentils with boiling water in a heavy-based pan, cover and cook for 20–30 minutes until tender. Drain and keep warm. Cover the mushrooms with boiling water and soak for 10–15 minutes to reconstitute them. Drain, and keep the liquid.

Put all the ingredients into a saucepan, and include the mushroom liquid, topping up with extra boiling water to just cover if necessary. Bring to the boil, turn down the heat and braise very gently for 30 minutes. Adjust the seasoning. Meanwhile, cook the bulgur by placing it in a pan, covering it with roughly three times its volume of boiling water, and cooking until the water is absorbed. Season well. In a small pan, cook the onion in the vegetable oil until it is well-browned but not blackened. Stir the onion into the bulgur, along with the marjoram and adjust the seasoning. Arrange the bulgur on plates and accompany with the lentil mixture.

Lentils baked with Almond Sauce

You could use either pecans or cashews for the sauce here. Almonds have more calcium in them than other nuts and also are a good source of vitamin E, B group vitamins and minerals such as zinc and iron.

4–5 fresh sage leaves
100g/4oz cooked lentils
100g/4oz cooked rice
25g/1oz cooked peas
4 tablespoons breadcrumbs
1 egg, beaten
50g/2oz ground almonds
3 tablespoons rolled oats
1 tablespoon sunflower seeds, finely ground
1 onion, finely sliced
4 tablespoons safflower or grapeseed oil
2 tablespoons tomato purée
2 plump cloves garlic, crushed
leaves from 1 sprig dried sage, finely sieved
salt & freshly ground black pepper

for the Almond Sauce:
500ml/16fl oz/2 cups water
75g/3oz whole peeled almonds
1 tablespoon tamari
1 tablespoon sesame oil
4 tablespoons parsley, finely chopped

Preheat the oven to 180°C/350°F/gas 4.

Mix all the ingredients for the bake in a large bowl and taste; adjust the seasoning. Line a loaf tin with the sage leaves and then spoon in the mixture. Bake in the oven for about 45 minutes, until nicely browned.

Make the sauce by putting all the ingredients except the parsley into a liquidiser and blitz until very smooth. Pour into a small pan and heat it over a medium flame until the mixture starts to thicken; stir the whole while.

Cut the lentil bake into slices and pour over some of the sauce, then sprinkle with parsley. Accompany with a crisp green salad made with a mixture of fresh leaves and a honey vinaigrette. Delicious!

RECIPES ON THIS AND THE FOLLOWING PAGES ALL SERVE 4 PEOPLE

Roasted Vegetables with Smoked Tofu

2 large red onions, sliced

3–4 fat cloves garlic, roughly chopped

4 large, well-flavoured tomatoes, such as Marmande, peeled and cut in half

2 large aubergines, cut into cubes

4 courgettes, cut into cubes

4 sweet red peppers, deseeded and cut into cubes

1 parsnip, scrubbed and cubed

6–8 tablespoons extra-virgin olive oil

a handful fresh basil leaves

500g/1lb smoked tofu, cut into cubes

sea salt & freshly ground black pepper

Heat the oven to 190°C/375°F/gas 5.

Put the onions, garlic, tomatoes (cut side down), aubergines, courgettes, peppers and parsnip into a large baking tin, drizzle over the olive oil and season with salt and pepper. Roast in the oven for 30 minutes until the vegetables are softened and just beginning to blacken. Add the tofu and basil leaves, and stir in well. Continue cooking for a further 15 minutes. Remove and serve, accompanied by bulgur wheat or a risotto made with brown rice.

Cauliflower & Mushrooms in Black Sauce

Taken from Rosamond Richardson's *Great Green Cookbook*, the cauliflower should be crunchy and is beautifully complimented by the black bean sauce.

1 tablespoon groundnut oil
350g/12oz cauliflower, broken into small florets
350g/12oz small button mushrooms, cut in half
2 cloves garlic, finely chopped
50g/2oz cashew nuts (unroasted)
2 tablespoons black bean sauce
2 tablespoons dark sesame oil
a handful of fresh coriander leaves to garnish

Heat the oil unti it smokes in a wok, then put in the cauliflower and mushrooms and stir-fry briskly until they are coated in the oil – about 1 minute. Then add the garlic and cashew nuts and sauté over a lower heat. Add 2 tablespoons of water, cover with a lid and steam until the cauliflower is tender – about 4–5 minutes.

Now stir in the black bean sauce and mix in well. Cover with a lid and warm through over a very low heat for a few minutes more.

Toss in the dark sesame oil just before serving, and garnish with a few fresh coriander leaves.

Broccoli & Tofu Stir-fry with Peanut Sauce

Tamari, made from soya beans, tastes salty and is available in health food stores. Use the best quality peanuts you can find; peanuts have the highest protein content of all nuts and are also provide plenty of vitamin B. This recipe is taken from *The Enchanted Broccoli Forest* by Mollie Katzen.

500g/1lb broccoli, broken up into small florets
4 tablespoons vegetable oil
2.5cm/1in ginger, peeled and grated
2 cloves garlic, crushed
2 tablespoons tamari
500g/1lb tofu, cubed
2 red onions, peeled and finely chopped
75g/3oz peanuts, crushed
spring onions to garnish

for the peanut sauce:
50g/2oz peanut butter
1 teaspoon coriander
1 teaspoon cumin
$\frac{1}{2}$ teaspoon honey
juice of 2 lemons
2 cloves garlic
6 tablespoons water
2 tablespoons tamari

Stir-fry the broccoli florets in a wok in a little of the oil, with the ginger and garlic until the broccoli is bright green and just tender. Stir in the tamari. Remove the pan and set aside.

Add a little more oil to the pan and stir-fry the tofu over a medium heat for 4–5 minutes. Add to the broccoli.

Add a little more oil to the pan and gently stir-fry the onions until they are soft. Add the peanuts to the onions and heat through.

Meanwhile, make the peanut sauce by whisking all the ingredients together in a small saucepan over a low heat until blended. Stir in sufficient water to make a thick creamy sauce.

Mix together the broccoli and tofu with the onions and peanuts and pour over the sauce, tossing gently over a low heat until well mixed. Serve over rice or pasta, sprinkled with the spring onions to garnish.

Winter Roasted Squash with Peanut Sauce

Increasingly we have a wider range of squashes to choose from. When roasted, squash takes on a smoky flavour and makes a warming vegetable. Peanuts grow underground and they are a good source of protein; use the best quality peanuts you can find. Serve with plenty of a good grain, such as quinoa. Quinoa is another great source of protein. It is cooked by adding a quantity of quinoa to double its quantity of water; boil for 15 minutes.

roughly 1kg/2lb various squashes
2 tablespoons olive oil
1 red onion, finely sliced
50g/2oz brown sugar
2 fresh red chillies, deseeded and finely chopped
1 tablespoon tahini
1 tablespoon peanut butter
400ml/14fl oz coconut milk
fresh coriander leaves, to garnish
salt & freshly ground black pepper

Preheat the oven to 200°C/400°F/gas 6.

Peel the squashes and cut into slices. Arrange on a lightly oiled baking tray and roast the squash in the oven until soft; this will take 20-30 minutes.

Make the sauce by heating the oil in a small, heavy-based pan and cooking the onion until it is softened. Add the sugar and chillies and stir constantly while the sugar melts. Then add the tahini and peanut butter and mix thoroughly, stirring all the time; dilute with the coconut milk and take care that the mixture doesn't stick to the bottom of the pan.

Arrange the squash on a bed of your chosen grain, season lightly to bring out the flavours, and pour over some of the sauce; garnish with coriander leaves

Spicy Potato Curry

350g/12oz potatoes, scrubbed
2 onions, peeled and finely sliced
4 tablespoons vegetable oil
1 tablespoon black mustard seeds
8–10 curry leaves
2 bot green chillies, very finely chopped
$\frac{1}{4}$ teaspoon turmeric
2 cloves garlic, finely crushed
2 teaspoons cumin seeds
2 teaspoons corriander seeds
1 tablespoon tomato paste disolved in a cup of boiling water
sea salt & freshly ground black pepper
coriander to garnish

Cook the cleaned potatoes in a large pan of boiling, salted water and drain. Keep the water in which they were cooked for later use. When cooled, cube the potatoes. Fry the onions in the vegetable oil until well-browned. Add the mustard seeds, and after a few seconds they will start popping. Then add the curry leaves. Add the potatoes, chillies, spices and finally the tomato paste and liquid, using the original potato water to cover the ingredients. Simmer for 10 minutes. Season and garnish with fresh coriander.

Side Dishes and Dips

Saffron Lentils

The Italians use small red lentils for this; after all the word 'lentil' is believed to have been taken from this protein-rich vegetable by Lentulus, one of the great Roman families. Soak the lentils for about 30 minutes before cooking.

3 tablespoons extra virgin olive oil
1 small red onion, finely chopped
2 bay leaves
300g/10oz/1½ cups red lentils
600ml/1pint vegetable stock
Several saffron strands
sea salt & freshly ground black pepper

Heat the olive oil in a heavy-based pan and add the onion and bay leaves. When the onion has softened, add the lentils and stir to coat with the oil. Add the vegetable stock and bring to the boil. Cover and cook for about 20-30 minutes. Season, and add the saffron, stirring to dissolve, and continue cooking until the liquid has all but evaporated. Discard the bay leaves and serve.

Braised Leeks

Slow, gentle braising keeps the full flavour of the leeks and makes them extremely tender and succulent. A dash of wine improves the dish no end.

4–6 leeks, depending on size, trimmed and washed
300ml/½ pint vegetable stock
2 tablespoons white wine
1 tablespoon fresh thyme leaves
sea salt & freshly ground black pepper

Preheat the oven to 190°C/375°F/gas 5.

Lay the leeks in a greased, oven-proof dish and pour over the stock. Sprinkle the thyme leaves over and season with salt and pepper. Cook in the oven for 40 minutes, until the leeks are soft when tested at the base end with a knife. Serve.

Guacamole

There are as many recipes for making this as there are for moussaka; everyone has their favourite one and this is mine. You can add chilli, sour cream or diced and peeled tomatoes; the flavours come through best when guacamole is served thoroughly chilled.

2 ripe avacados, mashed
juice of 1 lemon
2 shallots, finely chopped
2 plump cloves garlic, crushed
sea salt & freshly ground black pepper

Put all the ingredients into a bowl and mix thoroughly. Adjust the seasoning and serve immediately. Use with tortilla chips, chunks of wholemeal bread or as an accompaniment to dishes such as Lentil Bake with Almond Sauce (see page 136).

Wilted Greens

Young vegetable leaves are best for this; their fresh taste comes through and they are extremely nutritious. There's plenty to choose from – Swiss chard, spinach, sorrel, rocket, beetroot tops, carrot tops, broad bean tops...

2 tablespoons extra-virgin olive oil
$\frac{1}{2}$ red chilli, deseeded and finely chopped
2 cloves garlic, finely chopped
4–6 large handfuls of mixed greens
salt & freshly ground black pepper

Heat the oil in a heavy-based pan and add the chilli and garlic. Toss well to coat and then add the greens. Stir and cook very briefly until they wilt but remain crunchy – 15 seconds usually does the trick. Season and serve immediately.

Red Bean Dip

These legumes are rich in fibre, minerals and vitamins. Try not to store them for more than about six months or they begin to deteriorate. This simple, flavourful dip always goes down well.

100g/4oz/1 cup dried kidney beans
2 cloves garlic, crushed with a little salt
1 jalapeno pepper, deseeded
3 tablespoons water
5 tablespoons safflower oil
$1\frac{1}{2}$ tablespoons cider vinegar
$\frac{1}{4}$ teaspoon paprika
$\frac{1}{2}$ teaspoon chilli powder
salt & freshly ground black pepper

Cover the kidney beans with boiling water and soak for 12 hours, preferably overnight. Drain and put into a saucepan with clean water; bring to the boil and cover, simmering for 45 minutes to 1 hour, depending on how fresh the beans are.

Put the garlic and pepper into a blender and blitz for a couple of seconds. Then add the beans and slowly pour in the water and oil to make a smooth thick paste. Finally add the remaining ingredients. Blitz to ensure all is well mixed and adjust seasoning if necessary.

Puddings

Baked Peaches

Deliciously summery, the quality of the peaches is all-important in this dish. Yellow peaches have a sweeter taste generally and a slightly firmer texture, although the flavour of white peaches is superior.

6–8 peaches, depending on size
2 tablespoons lemon juice
2–3 tablespoons runny honey
$\frac{1}{2}$ teaspoon ground cinnamon
$\frac{1}{2}$ teaspoon grated nutmeg
$\frac{1}{2}$ teaspoon vanilla extract

Preheat the oven to 180°C/350°F/gas 4.

Pop the peaches into boiling water for a few seconds, Drain and remove their skins. Cut in half and remove the stones, then slice. Put them into a greased oven-proof dish and sprinkle over the spices, stirring gently. Bake in the oven for about 45 minutes. Serve either warm or cold.

Raisin & Hazelnut Pudding

You could use sultanas and almonds just as well in this warming winter pudding.

100g/4oz/⅔ cup cane sugar
25g/1oz margarine
100g/4oz/⅔ cup raisins
175ml/7fl oz boiling water
1 teaspoon vanilla extract

for the pudding:
75g/3oz/¾ cup whole wheat flour
1 teaspoon baking powder
4–6 tablespoons soya milk
a handful of hazelnuts, roughly chopped

Preheat the oven to 180°C/350°F/gas 4.

Put half each of the sugar and margarine into a small saucepan with the raisins and pour over the boiling water. Bring gently to the boil and cook at just simmering point for 5 minutes. Stir in the vanilla extract and set aside.

For the pudding, put the rest of the sugar and margarine into a food processor, together with the flour and baking powder. Blitz for a couple of seconds and then add enough soya milk to make a thick batter.

Pour the batter into a greased, oven-proof dish and add the raisin mixture. Stir once and sprinkle with nuts. Cook in the pre-heated oven for 40 minutes until risen and nicely browned. Serve immediately.

Plum Crumble

Made with oats, rather than white flour, this becomes a protein-rich pudding. Oat flour can be used as an alternative to wheat flour in dishes but will make them slightly heavier. Apples, prunes, pears can be used to ring the changes from plums.

750g/1½lb plums, such as Victorias, Early Rivers
1 teaspoon cinnamon
a little brown sugar (optional)
150g/6oz oats
75g/3oz wheat germ
75g/3oz desiccated coconut
75g/3oz soft brown sugar
5–6 tablespoons oil

Preheat the oven to 190°C/375°F/gas 5.

Cut the plums in half and remove the stones. Arrange the plums in greased, oven-proof dish and sprinkle with cinnamon and the sugar if desired.

Put the remaining ingredients into a food processor and blitz for a couple of seconds. Pour the crumble over the fruit and cook in the oven for 30–40 minutes. Serve.

Chapter 6
Exercise and structure

Posture

Posture is a very important part of the whole structural maintenance of the body. Poor posture can be responsible for both minor and major problems from backache to scoliosis and from headaches to digestive problems.

Everything we do during the course of the day determines how our postural muscles do or don't work effectively. To maintain the right spacing of the vertebrae of the spine and to allow sufficient room at each of these spaces for the nerve roots to spread out and create the nerves running all over the body, posture has to be maintained correctly.

The old victorian maxim of stand tall, walk tall and sit tall was very much based on the correct premise. All day long, gravity is squashing us in the process of holding us on the planet and if we consciously stretch ourselves out then we can maintain adequate space between the vertebrae for all the nerve functions to be normal. Leaning constantly to one side or the other, bending forward, rounding shoulders, arching the back or curving the spine when sitting in a slouched position are all parts of the lack of postural control which can lead to problems in the structural system.

Posture is not a static and rigid process but is one of being aware of how the body is being held, of standing straight, of stretching and making sure that whenever we sit we have support for the back or, if the chair is not suitable to sit on, with support, we can sit forward on the chair and use our back muscles to hold us in a correct position. It is always important to think of the quality of chairs used in the house, in the office and of equipment we use. We should also know how to use car seating effectively, and be aware of all the factors that affect how we control and support our posture, both by exercise and furniture and fittings during the day.

The Alexander Technique, mentioned in chapter four, is an excellent form of learning all about postural control.

Posture is very important in quality of exercise. For instance, walking, if carried out in a bad posture with rounded shoulders, can restrict breathing; a bent back prevents the leg muscles working effectively and freely and gives poor neck and head alignment. All these reduce the value of the walk to a considerable degree. The critical advice on the subject of posture is always to think of how we do whatever we have to do that relates to using the body during the course of the day. It is by not being aware of what the body is doing that many accidents occur and a lot of damage can be done to the structure as a whole.

Structure

The osteopath's tenet is that structure controls function; by this, they mean that if your body maintains a normal, balanced structure (muscles and joints), you will enjoy good health. Although this may be slightly exaggerated, there is no doubt that the spine is important on a whole, organic body level.

The spine is the mechanism that keeps the body functioning. It separates the pelvis and cranium; the positioning of the vertebrae affects how the nerves function and can cause either interference with the nerve function (generally felt as pain) or affect the function of organs when non-pain sensory nerves are affected.

To create and maintain health, the body's structure must be good. The spine must be aligned and in balance; this also affects the energy flow through the body, and the more the spine is out of alignment, the more problems you'll face.

Why we need exercise

Exercise and movement are part of life. The body is designed to move – it needs movement if it is to maintain muscle tone, which keeps the organs in the right place, which in turn keeps the circulatory system in place. For example, if you're overweight, the excess fat will affect your arteries and this will affect your body's ability to function normally. And with today's sedentary lifestyle, you're likely to spend a great deal of time at your desk, sitting in a car, bus or train, or in an armchair – none of which bear much relation to the human shape, and can cause the spine to become rigid and out of alignment.

Your abdominal organs – particularly your intestines – are maintained by your pelvic floor muscles and the front of your abdomen. Many 'women's problems' are caused by poor muscular tone; this gives rise to congestion and poor drainage in the abdomen, which contributes to the build-up of toxins and can have a detrimental effect on the ovaries and uterus. In men, poor muscular tone affects the blood supply to the testicles, which affects fertility. Abnormal circulation congestion is potentially a factor in cancer, either testicular or prostate in men or ovarian and uterine in women.

Poor muscle tone plus bad circulation and the obstructions we've mentioned before (nutritional and psychological) lead to lowered energy and lowered immune system – a major factor in cancer. If our intestines are not working properly and our muscle tone is poor, we may suffer from IBS and diverticulitis. The constant inflammation and irritation in the intestines increases the possibility of cancer.

The good news is that the obstruction caused by poor structure is reversible – poor muscle tone can be improved by sensible exercise. Remember that you need to be fit to exercise, not exercise to get fit, so keep exercise at a level with which your body is comfortable and increase it only gradually.

Sensible exercise

The best form of exercise is walking because this is what our bodies are designed to do. Walk as much as you can – at least 10–15 minutes a day; it's important to do this unencumbered by shopping, briefcases or anything heavy.

Other forms of exercise that can help are mobility exercises, done on a daily basis, to help avoid muscular and structural problems.

Cancer and exercise

If you have cancer, while you're having treatment and in the process of re-creating your health, you should not exercise very strongly because there simply isn't enough in your energy bank account to pay out huge cheques. It's better to do some restricted exercise on a regular basis; three lots of ten minutes is less draining than one lot of thirty minutes. It's best to exercise little and often and to spread out the exercise during the day. The logic is, if you spend a huge cheque from your energy bank on a thirty-five or forty-minute walk, your bank account is depleted just at the moment your body may need energy for its immune system – energy that won't be there, so the direct debit will bounce and slow down the body's progress.

There is a major interaction between exercise, nutrition and your emotional state (the three obstructions to normal function) and each can affect the other positively or negatively. For example, if we eat poor food then we develop poor quality muscle, which affects our ability to exercise. If we are not sufficiently mobile and don't get adequate exercise, then our circulation and the blood supply to our brains is adversely affected. This can make us more prone to stress and tension, which in turn creates muscular tension, to the extent that it interferes with the nerve supply to the digestion and, however good the food, digestion cannot be as effective as it should be. As we see, the body is a complete whole and posture and exercise are part of this equation of health.

On the positive side, taking regular exercise produces good muscular tone and circulation; this leads to good blood supply to the brain, the ability to use our mind more positively, less stress and greater well-being. As always, the body allows us to restore balance if we really take the appropriate steps.

A lot of the exercises I recommend are yoga-based; they're good for mobility. If you go to a yoga teacher, the mental and emotional philosophy behind the exercises work in harmony with the physical exercise to balance your body.

I recommend that the following programme of exercises is done morning and evening, to help increase mobility and fitness in a gentle way.

Starting to exercise

If you haven't done exercise before, start with gentle walking until you feel able to tackle something more, and then start with this programme. All the exercises should be repeated five times.

When you're recovering from cancer, remember that you'll have a low level of fitness. Go by how you feel; if you feel tired afterwards, you're overdoing it, so don't do so much next time. Do three repetitions instead, then work up steadily to five and keep within your comfort zone. You can maintain or re-create your health by listening to your body: when you're tired, your body wants to rest.

Hip circling (both ways)

With your feet comfortably apart, your hands on your hips and your knees unlocked, push your pelvic girdle in a complete circle in each direction. It's important not to lock your knees as your circle your hips, as this will prevent the range of movement you need to fully mobilise and exercise your lower back.

Side stretching

With your feet comfortably apart, your knees unlocked and your back straight, slide your left arm down your left leg while you curl your right arm across the top of the head, then repeat on the opposite side. Make sure you don't lean forward while you're doing this exercise. In the upright position, stretching to the side mobilises the spine in the upright position, which means that it spaces the vertebrae equally in the process of applying the stretch, and the muscles are working in their proper postural alignment. By leaning forward, we stretch the vertebrae unevenly and out of alignment, and are encouraging abnormal muscle pulls in the whole process.

Neck stretch

Stretch your neck over to your right side and try to increase the movement by letting the restraining muscles relax; this will let your head move over as far to the side as possible. Repeat on the left side. Stretch your chin towards your chest – again, relaxing the controlling muscles to let your head move forward as far as possible – and then slowly move your head back upright and let it drop back, using the weight of your head as the stretching mechanism. Finally, starting with your chin to the right, let your head roll in a semi-circle across the front of your body and finish on the left. Repeat with your head dropped back, but don't take your head in a full circle or you'll cause discomfort in your neck.

Shrugging

Pull your shoulders up as close to your ears as possible, then rotate them in a full circle, first of all moving forwards for a complete circuit and then backwards for a complete circuit.

Cat stretch

Kneel with your knees together and place your hands on the floor at right-angles to your body, shoulder-width apart, with your back straight. Bend your head down and arch your back fully upwards. In a gradual and controlled movement, extend your head up and let your spine sag down as far as it can go without undue pressure. As your mobility improves, you can start to increase the pressure in both directions.

Kneeling press-ups

Kneel with your knees together and place your hands on the floor at right-angles to your body, shoulder-width apart, with your back straight and your face looking down. Bend your arms until your face is lowered to the floor, then straighten again to raise your body to the original position. Keep your legs still throughout the exercise, as it is designed to increase mobility around your hips.

Abdominal press

Lie on your back with your knees bent and your feet flat on the ground. Breathe out and flatten your whole spine as much as possible against the floor. Hold this position for 10 seconds and then relax and let your spine come away from the floor.

Increasing the amount you exercise

Once you've mastered the basic exercises, increase your morning and evening routine to include the following, all at five repetitions each:

Hip circling (both ways)
As above

Side stretching
As above

Trunk twisting (both ways)
With your feet comfortably apart, your hands on your hips and your knees unlocked, circle your body above your waist in a complete movement in both directions. Do not lock your knees or you will strain your lower back.

Arm stretch
Stand up straight with your legs together and your arms straight out in front of you, with your thumbs just touching. Move your whole shoulder girdle in a complete arc in each direction; make this movement as full as possible to improve your mobility in the neck and shoulder area.

Neck stretch
As above

Shrugging
As above

Arm swinging

Stand upright with your knees slightly bent. Swing your right arm up and forward, scraping your ear on the way past, and swing around the back as far as possible. Repeat with the left arm. Ensure the swing is as full as possible and don't move the rest of your body while you exercise your arms. Then swing both arms forward and up in a full circle, then back and up in a full circle.

Cat stretch

As above

Forehead to knee (alternate)

Kneel with your knees together and place your hands on the floor at right-angles to your body, shoulder-width apart, with your back straight. Bend your head between your arms and bring your right knee towards the forehead, as far as you can without feeling uncomfortable. Lift your head and bring your knee back to the floor, then repeat with your left knee. When you first do this exercise, you may find a large gap between your knee and forehead, but this will diminish steadily as the mobility of your spine increases.

Opposite arm and leg stretch

Kneel with your knees together and place your hands on the floor at right-angles to your body, shoulder-width apart, with your back straight. Stretch out your left arm and right leg, and stretch out your head and neck slightly upwards. Bring your arm and leg back to the starting point and repeat with your right arm and left leg. As your body becomes fitter and stronger, you will be able to hold the stretch for a longer period and stretch out further.

Hip stretch

Sit with your left leg stretched straight out in front of you and your right knee bent with your heel flat on the floor and close to your body. Gradually stretch your right knee down to the floor at the side until your leg is flat against the floor – you won't be able to stretch that far at first but with time and effort you'll manage it. Repeat with the other leg.

Kneeling press-ups

As above

Abdominal press

As above

Alternate knee raises

Lie on your back with your legs straight out in front of you and your arms by your sides. Raise your left knee towards your chest, then let it go back to its original position and repeat with your right knee.

If you're used to exercise

Where sport and high activity are concerned, only play sport if you are fit, rather than playing to improve your fitness. If you're fit, then the exercise is beneficial and you're less likely to injure yourself; otherwise, you're writing out huge energy cheques and there's nothing to pay out. Just think of the archetypal unfit person having a heart attack on the squash court – it's important to be fit first.

If you play sport regularly and are used to exercise, use the following routine morning and night.

Hip circling (both ways)
As above – 5 repetitions

Side stretching
As above – 5 repetitions

Trunk twisting (both ways)
As above – 5 repetitions

Arm stretch
As above – 5 repetitions

Neck stretch
As above – 5 repetitions

Shrugging
As above – 5 repetitions

Arm swinging
As above – 5 repetitions

Cat stretch
As above – 10 repetitions

Forehead to knee (alternate)
As above – 10 repetitions

Opposite arm and leg stretch
As above – 10 repetitions

Sit-ups to alternate knee

5 repetitions. Lie on your back with your hands behind your neck. Raise your left knee towards the midpoint of your body and lift your head and shoulders at the same time. Lower your knee, head and shoulders and repeat with the right knee. As your strength and mobility increases, your knee and head will come nearer together and you will be able to hold the position for longer. Take care with both these sit-ups, particularly in the early stage, that you don't over-stretch and strain your neck.

Sit-ups to both knees

5 repetitions. Lie on your back with your hands behind your head and your knees bent. Curl up gradually and bring your forehead towards your knees. Even if you can't lift up fully at first, time and perseverance will help.

Hip stretch

As above – 10 repetitions

Kneeling press-ups

As above – 10 repetitions

Abdominal press

As above – 10 repetitions

Chest raises/leg lifts

10 repetitions. Lie down flat on your stomach with your hands behind your neck. Relax, then raise your upper trunk, bringing your elbows up, raising your head and neck backwards and creating as much of an arch as possible. Hold the position for a moment, relax to the starting position, and repeat.

Then raise your legs upwards as far as possible, without lifting your trunk. Hold for a few moments, lower your legs, relax and repeat. As your body tone improves, you will be able to arch further and hold the position for longer

Alternate knee raises
As above – 10 repetitions

Breathing exercises

Breathing exercises are an important part of exercise. I've already mentioned that yoga is particularly beneficial, in a combination of breathing and gentle stretching exercises to help destress you.

The breathing process increases the oxygenation of your blood and works your diaphragm. This in turn works your stomach muscles and solar plexus, the base of your ribcage and your abdomen. It's important to focus on the outbreath; however much oxygen you get into your lungs on the inbreath, it can't be absorbed until the carbon dioxide has been filtered out of your blood. If you've ever given anyone the kiss of life, you'll know that the first breath of a resuscitated person is the outbreath, and the body takes over from there.

If you breathe out properly, you're using your lungs properly. This means that your whole ribcage will move when you breathe, and the process of breathing will remove any rubbish from the base of your lungs and enable oxygen to be absorbed more easily.

The lungs are like a bellows; practice your breathing by expanding the base of your ribcage and your diaphragm simultaneously. With the outbreath, contract your ribcage and diaphragm. The aim is to get as much movement as possible in the body; it will increase with practice as your lungs become more efficient. Yoga can be very beneficial as breathing exercises are a specific part of the programme.

Sex

Sexual intercourse is only one part of a loving relationship. Remember that it has a high energy output and view it in the light of your other activities during the day. The rule has to be that if you want to do it and you feel able to do it, then it will not hurt you.

Chapter 7
Psychological, emotional and spiritual matters

The psychological, emotional and spiritual obstructions to energy can be very draining. If we have a negative outlook on life, then psychologically we're setting ourselves up to fail at what we try to do; emotionally, we'll feel bad; and we may feel very alone and remote from any spiritual comfort.

One of the biggest problems is the habit of looking to the future instead of living in the present. Looking forward to the future is never a helpful process. In the present, we may plan for the future but should remember that those plans may or may not mature, dependent upon what we actually do in the present as it unfolds. Having made a plan, we should then leave it to mature or otherwise in the passage of life itself and act upon what happens when it happens.

Many people spend months looking *forward* to a holiday, a special occasion or an event of note. While looking forward with pleasure is at least positive, unfortunately it does nothing to create or change anything in the present. Anticipation can often be misleading and indeed can lead to disappointment. The Bible says 'blessed is he who expecteth nothing, for he shall not be disappointed' and, while that is true, more significantly, if we live fully in the *present* we do not need to expect anything.

Fear

Looking forward with fear is one of the major causes of severe stress and tension; mentally, emotionally and spiritually. We have all lived through many situations where we have lost sleep, being severely worried and very unhappy about something we expect to happen in the future. Frequently, the event we worry about never happens at all, or when it happens there is something that can be done to deal with it or it is of much less significance than we anticipated.

There is a wonderful story taken from *The Eyes of Horus* by Joan Grant (second edition by Ariel Press, 1988), a book about the education of a young pharaoh-to-be in ancient Egypt.

The story tells of a prince who was seeking adventure travelling the world. He came upon a village at the bottom of two mountains with a valley in between. On top of one of the mountains was a huge fire and a smoke-breathing dragon. When the prince reached the village everybody was sad, crying, wailing or just sitting down despondently. He spoke to the head man of the village saying, 'What is the matter? Why are you all so sad and depressed?'

The head man replied. 'It is because of the dragon. Our fields where all our crops are grown are on the other side of the valley and, because the dragon is so big, and breathes so much smoke and fire down into the valley, we cannot pass through to reach our crops. We have very little food left now; we are too far from anywhere to go to find food; and soon we shall all die of starvation.'

The prince said, 'Has no one tried to fight the dragon? At least that way you would have a chance of ridding yourself of this menace.'

The head man replied, 'Our bravest man tried last week and started up the mountain to try to kill to the dragon. Unfortunately, the path is so narrow and so strewn with loose rocks that he fell to his death before he was able to tackle the dragon and fight him. The day before yesterday, the only other man in our village who knows how to use the sword said that he would try, but unfortunately the same fate befell him and we now have no one else left who would have any chance of defending us against this dragon.'

'Then I must try and fight the dragon for you,' said the prince, and put on his armour and took out his sword.

When the prince reached the bottom of the mountain, he was well aware of the dragon roaring above and saw how narrow and stony the path was that led up the mountain. He decided that the one thing he would not do was fall off the path, so at least if he died he would die fighting the dragon and not from slipping. As he started up the mountain, he looked carefully where he was putting each foot and he moved loose stones out of the way and went slowly up the steep path. He paused for a breath or two of deep air and, looking around him, saw the beautiful view down to the valley below and at the same time noticed where one of his predecessors had fallen, which made him even more determined to be careful of the path.

He continued upwards, pausing periodically to take a breath and to look at the view in front of him, and then continued carefully past where the other brave man from the village had fallen, picking his way up the path. After a period of time, to his surprise, he found himself standing on top of the mountain and found that he could not see the dragon anywhere. He called challengingly and heard a squeak by his feet. He bent down and picked up a small creature, which turned out to be a tiny dragon.

'Where is your big brother?' said the prince. 'I have come here to fight him to save the lives of the villagers below.'

'There is only me here,' said the tiny dragon.

To which the prince responded, 'How can this be, that such a tiny dragon as you can cause so much terror and fear in the hearts of so many people?'

'That's easy,' said the dragon. 'I can do that because of my name.'

'What is your name?' said the prince.

The dragon said, 'My name is What Might Happen.'

From a distance, what might happen looks terrifying. The fear of what might happen changes how people act in the present and can lead to many – and even fatal – errors on the way. By concentrating on the path to the future, i.e. the present, when we reach 'What Might Happen', it is still a dragon, but one that can be picked up in the palm of the hand.

Living in the present

This story very clearly explains how living in the present can create a future which, even if it does have the odd dragon, can be coped with in a positive, constructive and productive manner. Whenever we feel fears and worries and find ourselves getting emotionally stressed, we should ask, 'What am I afraid of?', 'What am I stressed about?', and 'Where is it?'

If it is not in the present, then all we need to do is to put it to the future where it belongs and do something constructive in the present: just looking around at the sun or flowers or anything which is part of life itself is sufficient to create a positive change and bring us back into the reality of what is in front of us.

Using the mind positively

Using the mind positively is fundamental to the process of learning to deal with any problems in life and, indeed, even life itself, but it becomes of paramount importance when you are faced with cancer. Cancer is a word which creates instant fear and stress in the life of anybody who has a suggestion of a diagnosis or an actual diagnosis of being a sufferer. People are afraid to discuss the condition, mention the name or even talk about it to people who are suffering from it or who have suffered from it.

Fear itself is in fact, one of the major factors in creating the fertile environment for the cancerous growth. Indeed, there is a lot of anecdotal evidence to suggest that, in many cases, where no diagnosis has been made, the fear of contracting and suffering from cancer can be a major factor in making sure that this actually comes to pass. The power of the mind is infinite and fear is just as strong as positivity and creativity in its influence on the mind.

The way we say or think about things can make a huge difference. You are only restricted by your level of belief – and there's a quick test to demonstrate the effectiveness of the power of words. Ask someone to face you and squeeze their thumb and forefinger together. Tell them to say, 'I will try to hold my finger and thumb together.' Try to pull their finger and thumb apart, and you'll find that you can separate them easily. Try the same trick again, but this time tell them to say, 'I will hold my finger and thumb together.' And, this time, you won't be able to separate their finger and thumb easily. The difference between *try* and *will* totally changes the body's self-belief and energy.

Viewing everything for the best

To use the mind positively means that we have to look upon everything and see the best in it; the old example of the glass which is half-empty to the pessimist and half-full to the optimist is a very good object lesson. The more we make positive decisions to view everything for the best, the easier it will become and the more we will find ourselves doing this naturally.

Sadly, it applies equally to negativity. The world today is very negative and all the news that we see, read or hear tends to be bad. There are wars, starvation and murders almost everywhere we look and because of this it is very easy to get sucked into the negative thinking mode. To avoid this, the critical thing that we have to do – and the only true positivity – is to learn to love and respect ourselves, and always do our best to deal positively with what is actually in front of us.

Love

Love is a much used and abused word in the English language and has come to take on a number of meanings. True love should always be unconditional and is the basis of all effective human relationships. If we love ourselves and, indeed, respect ourselves, then we can love and respect other people; but if we do not have this inner love, then it is almost impossible to love someone else without there being a whole series of conditions and restraints on the love that we give.

Our relationship with others is an integral part of building a positive and constructive world for ourselves. If we can not interrelate lovingly and happily with the people around us, it is impossible to maintain a level of well-being, on the physical, mental and spiritual levels, that is necessary to maintain real health.

Starting within ourselves

To be positive, the only place to start is within ourselves and by creating personal positivity we will affect others around us with equal positivity. We have all met someone who makes us feel exhausted when we've talked to them for a quarter of an hour – this is the negative – and equally we have all met someone who makes us feel totally energised and elated when we've spent half an hour together. The choice of which kind of person we want to be is entirely our own.

Initially, it is often quite hard work to develop the concept of looking for the good in everybody and everything, but it becomes progressively much easier with the realisation that there truly is good in everything and everybody. It is a wonderful experience to recognise this. With this change in approach to ourselves and thus to other people, we also can develop the necessary change in how we think about our health. This is a very important part of the procedure of creating and maintaining health.

The people around us

The last part of maintaining the constructive mental and spiritual approach is to look at how we relate to people around us. I have already mentioned unconditional love, and in our relationships with other people it is also equally true that the only person who can make or spoil that relationship is ourself. We all have a tendency – which civilisation has encouraged – to take people for what they do, not for what they are. This, of course, leads to disappointment if people do not do what we think they should do or what we would expect them to do because of what we have done.

Looking at it realistically, of course, this is impossible to maintain effectively as the only person that we control is ourself, and we cannot have any direct effect upon what other people do. Nobody can make us happy, angry, sad, elated: we make ourselves all of these, depending upon how we decide to act upon the input from another person. We do not react to people, we act upon what they present to us. This means that we can decide whether to be happy, sad, angry or elated; these decisions are not made for us by somebody else.

Many of us tend to give out love like a present: here's a packet of love and, of course, I expect a packet of love back when it's my birthday or a favour returned for a favour done. This, unfortunately, creates a huge load of transfer of responsibility to another person by putting expectations upon them which are not truly reasonable.

If we make a decision to love somebody, to do something for somebody or to give something to somebody, this should be done from the position of it being what we want to do, what we believe we should do and, therefore, what we will do without any conditional restraints upon the transfer. If a gift is given in this fashion – and the gift can be material or spiritual – then the benefit to us has occurred at the moment of passing the gift over. What happens to it then is entirely up to the person to whom it is given, who will make their own choices in relation to who they are at the particular time in the present. The giving of the gift without conditions is the positive and constructive activity from our own point of view. We are responsible for our actions, not the results.

We have all heard many people say, 'Can you believe that, after all I have done for them?' and in honesty we have probably said it ourselves on many occasions as well. This of course is where we put on to the recipient of the gift a requirement to satisfy something within us in return.

Life does not work like this.

Whatever we put into life will determine what we get out of it. What we should put into life is everything that we can do positively at every moment of our existence in the present and do everything with love, with happiness and with no conditions. If we can achieve this, then life will bring to us everything that we need – not always (in fact, often rarely) from the place where the gift has been given, but always when it is needed from a place which is probably yet unknown to us.

The old Biblical saying 'as we sow, so we reap' is a very difficult fact to argue against. From the point of view of raising the energy and awareness levels of the mind, body and spirit of the human individual, the ability to release our fears, our expectations and our negativity are the roots of creating a totally healthy and functional body-mind-spirit entity.

The remarkable thing about something like cancer is that there are many people who, having been faced with cancer – either personally or through close friends and family – have found that it is a crisis which unlocks the door to a totally different way of life. A crisis is only a turning point and what nature can do, given the right environment, is in many cases truly miraculous.

We can achieve anything; all we have to do is to remove the obstructions to this process. Our use of our mind is a major step on the journey from fear, sickness and ill-health to releasing, from within ourselves, health, happiness and peaceful harmony.

De-stressing techniques

Finding out you have cancer can be extremely stressful. Stress itself is one of the causes of cancer; so beginning to remove the stress in your life will start the removal of another obstruction to getting well again. Many people find they need help with this, and a common starting point is with counselling – choose a practitioner who is qualified, who has specialised in the management of stress and who creates positivity rather than assigning blame.

Eeman technique

The Eeman technique is one that I've used for years to help this situation. Any mental or emotional stress or trauma creates a physical muscle tension – in other words, you feel uptight. The tension stays there. If the stress is repeated, the tension becomes stronger, and you therefore become more vulnerable to some types of stress or trauma. This creates a vicious circle which the Eeman technique can help to break.

The practitioner will go through your body, finding your unconscious tensions and teaching you how to relax these by movement and breathing techniques. He or she will then link one hand with yours on your solar plexus and another on your forehead, to increase your body's energy flow, helping further relaxation and releasing tension and trauma from your subconscious mind. This makes you less vulnerable to a repetition of the stress process and releases key held fears and trauma.

Thinking about what you do as you do it

The Alexander technique (see complementary therapy on page 79) is a postural awareness technique that teaches you to use your body positively and draws attention to any lack of conscious awareness which leads to mis-use and related problems of the structure of your body. If you don't think about what you're doing, you'll do them badly. I've shown this with a simple stage trick during lectures. I came onto the stage with what I said was a heavy suitcase – though it was actually empty – and asked for a strong member of the audience to help me. The person offering help usually flexes his muscles and thinks about how heavy the suitcase is going to be, rather than focusing on the task in question – so he always trips on the steps, then grabs the case and it flies in the air because it isn't as heavy as he's expecting. This may look funny, but it is a potential disaster.

The correct way to do it is to concentrate on getting onto the stage, watching as you go, and waiting until you reach the problem – the suitcase. Bend your knees, take a grip on the suitcase and straighten your knees and increase the strength of your grip until the suitcase leaves the floor. This is smooth, will not tear muscles if the case is very heavy, and only the necessary energy will be used. The idea is to use the least possible expenditure of energy for the maximum possible effect. If you're aware of your body and are at one with it, you'll be able to achieve great things. If you lose touch mentally with your body, you'll waste energy, get stiff and tense and become negative.

Other techniques

Many of the complementary therapies mentioned in Chapter 4 can also help with destressing and relaxation. Aromatherapy, Bach Flower Remedies, colour therapy, massage, reflexology and yoga are particularly good. This is because they allow you to spend time on yourself and not feel guilty about it; they allow you to concentrate on something else other than the problem that's worrying you, and also because of the physical effects of the treatments. As with all complementary treatments, it's best to consult a qualified practitioner or teacher to get the optimum results. Appendix 1 gives a list of organisations that can put you in touch with your nearest qualified practitioner.

Spiritual matters

Religion can be a difficult area for many people. Some religions have their own problems, such as Jehovah's Witnesses where the patient's treatment is limited by a prohibition on blood exchanges or extraction, and others such as Judaism where there are particular eating codes at various times. But all religions can be a huge help when used in a positive fashion.

It's important to have a belief in a greater power, whatever it may be called, and to understand that all religions almost universally have a basis of love and peace and harmony. In the interpretation of the original scriptures of these religions, this is often lost, but this is not the fault of the religions themselves where the interpretation can be misleading.

A family that has a united faith and a belief in the oneness of life is almost always of great support and comfort during times of crisis. Usually, people who practise religion positively and lovingly have a circle of friends of similar inclinations who can also be of great help and support when difficulties arise. Some religions, such as Seventh Day Adventists, have views about food which are similar to naturopathy, and this can be a great help.

Religion doesn't have to be organised. It can be one person – you – as all things are personal. I believe that religion can help to uplift and motivate people to find out more about who they are and would like to be, and when this happens it is a wonderful part of the health-maintenance programme.

Chapter 8
The whole person and cancer

Peter Wallace, the ex-chair of the *Bristol Cancer Help Centre*, has a lot to say on the subject we discussed in the last chapter – how we can help recover from cancer with the help of emotional, physical and spiritual lessons.

Cancer Help Centre lessons

I had the privilege of being asked to take on the role of Chairman on the *Bristol Cancer Help Centre* between 1994 and 1998. By then I had lost some dear friends to cancer, and I was interested in how healing of the whole person might work, so I accepted. I met some wonderful people during my time there, who taught me so much in different ways about the fear associated with cancer, both for the poor doctors who have to give the bad news, and the patients who are put into a state of often terminal shock.

I also learned two very important lessons about healing and cancer. The first is that it is very difficult for anyone to be involved in a charity that is based on loving support when you have to worry about where the next money for upkeep and wages of the staff are coming from. It detracts so much from the healing support that is needed. We need a better way of supporting places like Bristol.

Secondly, I learned that those who succeed in beating cancer seem to have one prevailing train. They take their life back, and make a conscious decision to live their life their way, and not as they think others want them to. They learn to be more of themselves, and to like themselves enough to allow themselves to be who they really are. In every moment, all the time, with everyone, every day.

Cancer people are wonderful people

People who get cancer, in my experience, are the nicest people you could ever hope to meet. They will do anything for anyone, and invariably they do! They will always see what needs to be done and quietly do it. They rarely make a fuss. They are wonderfully helpful and kind people to everyone.

The one person they tend to forget about is themselves

We are all connected

From as far back as I can remember in my life I have always had a question that needed an answer. 'Why do people have to get ill?' I would like to share with you, as my contribution to the cancer journey, what I have found.

I believe we are all connected to each other, as part of the whole that has created us. To me it seems that we are like the cells in the body. Each cell – a lung, heart, brain, foot, hand cell and so forth – has a role in the body, and is both a part of the body and an individual in its own right. Each cell's role is important to the healthy functioning of the whole body. Each cell has a purpose, or plan, or promise that it was created to fulfil. Each cell is both the body and a part of the body. We know from DNA that the plan for the whole body is in each cell!

We are no different. We are all parts of God, and so we are God too. You are God, here in your version of God's energy, here to express the particular aspect of God that you represent. This makes you very important, as well as everyone else.

So if we are to fulfil our individual plan for being here – whether it is to be the best mother, the best cake-maker, or the most creative gardener we can be – we have to give ourselves a chance.

It is time to choose for you what you need

Choosing for you

After spending so much time looking after others' needs, it may seem a little strange to try to remember who you really are and what you would like to do. You are looking for that part of you that makes you feel really whole and complete. That thing you can do you feel passionate about, that fills you with joy when you do it and think about doing it.

Each of us has our aspect of God that we are here to be. We can experience the joy of being this aspect of God on earth.

You may say now, 'How does all of this work? How can I make these connections with the real me again? I am frightened, I am full of the fear of death, I am in pain, I am worried about my family and friends, and I can't sleep easily at night.'

You are not alone

Remember you are not alone.

As part of the whole, you are connected to the whole

It is time to remember who you are and that you are not alone. Each of us has a voice inside – our conscience, our intuition, a feeling we get – that is there to guide us. Often we ignore it as not being realistic or relevant, but it is this part of us that we need to learn to listen to again.

For me, this voice is the God part of me – the Godself, the higher self, the guardian angel that looks after me. However we choose to see it, it is a part of us. And, like all good friends, it doesn't impose itself on you. I will call it our angel, from now on, for this is how most of us best accept this aspect of heaven that works with us.

Your angel and everyone else's angel can work with you

Ask and listen

You have to ask. They are with you all the time. As part of your plan in coming here, you agreed to take on the human role, and they agreed to be your angel. But they can do nothing unless you ask them for help. Ask as often as you like. Every moment of every day, if you like. It is a practical process of you asking – doing your best to trust that you are heard, for you are – and then listening to what you hear.

Listening is what we need to do most

Both with our friends on earth and our friends we can't see. I learned to listen by writing in a free way – asking a question and then writing what came into my mind. I learned through this to see the human answers and the angel answers. And the angel answers were so helpful to me.

This is what I found out about the answers I got.

Human answers always want to control a situation. They always want things to be the way we think they should be. They usually want someone else to change, and not us. Angel answers can never harm anyone, they leave everyone total freedom of choice, and work with love always to achieve a goal. By applying these simple tests you will quickly learn to distinguish between heaven (angel) and earth (human) answers.

Simply put, love sets you free, while fear tries to control and manipulate the situation in some way.

A loving environment

So you have a plan, that you share with an angel, which is what you came here to do. If you ask, you can get help with every situation you are in as you learn to listen to the answers that are there for you. The angels help by creating a loving environment around you, or the person you ask for help for. Most of us are a little stuck in our thinking, and this loving energy helps us to have more loving choices to choose from. We can still choose the less loving, more fearful route, but the angels help us feel that there is a bigger range of choices. This is their job, and their agreement with us.

Try asking now, when you are in a quiet space, 'What are you, my angel, trying to help me see with my cancer?' For you have chosen this route at this stage for a reason. It may be to get others to help you, it may be to get you to do more for yourself, it may be that you have finished what you came to do, or it may be that you are at the start of a new phase in your life. All of these reasons, and many more, are just some of the reasons we may choose cancer to help us move closer to love.

Cancer is never a judgement on you. It is a choice you and your angel make for you as part of your journey to love. Whichever choice you make, you will find the love that is you, If you choose to go home (to heaven) you will experience the joy of all of who you are, and if you choose to stay for a while longer, you will find the love of expressing more of you on earth.

Either way you will find the joy that is you

Nothing happens by chance

There is an important point in this understanding of life.

Nothing in life happens by chance. Everything happens to help you find more of the love that you are

This is why we choose the things that happen, to help us shake off the fear and choices we no longer want to make.

If we accept that possibility, and consider that there is some good to find in what we are experiencing, then we will find it. We always find what we look for, so choose carefully what you see in all that happens to you. As you allow the love that is you – the God that is you – to be expressed, you will begin to see how we always bring to ourselves situations that help us move towards love. No matter how difficult it might at first seem.

This is because everyone we are with is involved in our plan

Each of us, as God, is creating the reality that we are experiencing on behalf of the whole body that is the planet earth we live on. As we find the love within us in each situation we are in – as we choose love, which is our universal self, we will find we see more clearly what we can do with love together.

How does all this happen? How can we be creating our own reality each day? Surely it all happens by chance? How can there be a plan in it?

World traditions of reflection

All traditions around the world encourage reflection and prayer at night, and an *opening up to the world* process in the morning, This is because at night, while we sleep, the love that is us is more able to come into us. We meet on higher planes, with each other, with those who have left earth like our angels and departed friends, and we discuss how to move things on the next day.

As God – that part of God that we are – we create with others, who are also God, how we are going to learn to experience more love on earth. We choose the outline experiences of the next day. Maybe someone is going to be difficult with you to help you see how love can heal such a situation. Maybe by helping the person see a better way, or maybe by bringing out a frustration (a lack of love to heal) in you. For love does heal all.

So we keep experiencing different situations to help us see how love really works in life. We choose with our friends to keep repeating an experience until we get the loving message and act on it!

So our friends, both on earth, and in heaven as angels, help us to experience what we think will best help us to move on. We do this by experiencing how love will sort out the problem. We learn to ask questions like, 'What would love do now?' with each situation we encounter. We make an active choice more consciously to ourselves, either by controlling fear or freeing up love, to solve our issues in life.

So we create our own reality. We are that wonderful and that amazing, and we create reality with each other in a shared way. And we learn that the only way we can ever progress together is by one simple process.

Sharing love. Sharing who we are, which is love, with each other. And in this process we learn with each other who we are, who we want to be, what we want to let go of, and what we choose to bring to us.

Ask a friend to help by listening to you
Talk to a friend, Open the deepest part of your heart you can find to your friend, Ask them just to listen to you, please. You don't need their advice

unless you ask for it; you just need them to hear you saying who you are, and who you want to be, with them listening. This is how they can really help you. Listening to all of you. Then you can find out who you really are, and become more of this, more and more every day.

And you will see that this is a process for well-being. It is a way of helping you feel easy with life, It is how you begin to let go of disease – dis-ease. It is a way of living that frees everyone, including you, and is part of this changing age that we have chosen to be here to enjoy.

So what will help you on your journey through cancer will also help others to not even have to make your journey.

You will show them, through the freedom you allow yourself, more of you

You show that you have chosen to live freely, all of you. And if you choose not to change anything, having taken a look at it all, that really is fine too. Sometimes it is simply time to go home, to say goodbye, thank you for being a part of my living experience and to set everyone free by forgiving all that you may think they have done.

Enjoy your remaining time by setting everyone else, as well as yourself, free, knowing that you have chosen to go home to experience being all of you, rather than staying here to experience it.

Enjoy your choices
Enjoy the choices you make for you, know that it is all perfect, and that you are beginning to see how it all works. Remember that you are an amazing being of love and light, and that there is nothing you can't do once you have allowed the love that is you to become all of you. Everything that you have ever done that you regret was simply an experience of life to help you find love. Nothing more or less

If you think you have hurt someone, then tell them you are sorry for any hurt you have imposed. If you think someone has hurt you, then know that all that happened was that they missed a shared experience in using love effectively, and maybe next time it will be fine.

Love them unconditionally, and they will be healed in time enough to learn to love you

Life is a wonderful journey that we each choose to experience. We are here to have fun and to enjoy being that loving aspect of God that we each are. Fun, happiness and joy are your birthright, when you are ready to embrace more of who you really are. May all God's love, which is also your love, be with you!

Postscript
Finally, I would like to add that it is very important to feed your physical body well, too, as you make these emotional and spiritual changes on your cancer journey, extra nourishment from good food and/or good supplements will help you on this journey, giving a little more physical strength to cope with the medical and other healing choices you make for you.

Remember, whatever healing choices you make, embrace them with all of you, When you join in with others in your healing it becomes so much more powerful. Ask your angel which is the best way for you, and try to listen to what you hear as best you can. Ask friends what they think they would do in your circumstances. Sometimes they can offer you insights you may not have. Remember, they may well be a part of your plan!

Be happy, be love, be you

Chapter 9
Managing cancer and the re-creation of health

Dealing with cancer and the re-creation of your health is something that needs good management. Just as you manage your bank account each month, make sure that you have enough coming in to pay the bills and that the bills get paid, so you can manage your health, and make sure that you increase the income into your energy bank and decrease the expenditure.

We have already seen that ENERGY equals LIFE ENERGY minus OBSTRUCTIONS; the energy is then paid into the energy bank account.

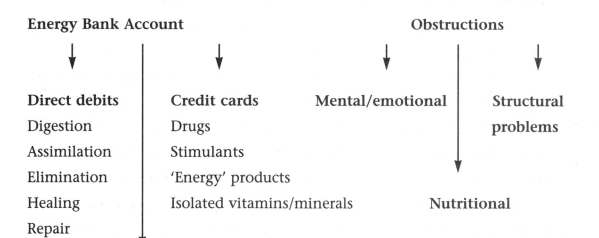

Energy Bank Account   **Obstructions**

Direct debits   **Credit cards**   **Mental/emotional**   **Structural**
Digestion   Drugs   **problems**
Assimilation   Stimulants
Elimination   'Energy' products
Healing   Isolated vitamins/minerals   **Nutritional**
Repair

Cheques
40% immediate increase when eyes are open
plus all conscious activities

Increasing your energy income

Increasing your energy income means removing the obstructions. And that means proper management of three key areas in your life: nutritional, structural and mental/emotional.

Nutritional

As we've already discussed, you need to put the best possible nutritional energy into your body – that means organic food, preferably locally produced, that has not been subjected to lengthy shipping or contamination from packaging. Raw or lightly cooked food is best; but because the vitamin and mineral content of foods has declined sharply over the last sixty years you'll also need to supplement your diet with food state nutrients, which give your body the choice of the nutrients it needs in the form most suitable for it. Eating three balanced meals a day will help your digestive system assimilate the food with the minimum amount of energy.

Structural

In addition to eating well, you need to pay attention to the way you use your body. Good posture will help your muscles work more effectively: that means standing tall, sitting with proper support and being aware of your movements when you exercise. Regular, appropriate exercise – such as walking and mobility exercises – will help to maintain your muscle tone, which in turn will keep your organs in the right place and maintain your circulatory system. When your body's structure is functioning properly, your energy levels will increase. It will also help you breathe properly – which in turn will help your body use oxygen more efficiently and remove the rubbish from your bloodstream.

Emotional

The power of the mind is often underestimated. If you worry all the time about the future – particularly about 'what might happen' – you're increasing stress and tension, which will affect your immune system and undermine your health. If you live in the present, you'll put things in their proper perspective and help yourself deal with any problems in a constructive, positive and productive way.

Looking at things positively and seeking the good in everyone and everything will help you think about the positive creation of health. Be responsible for your own actions and learn to love others unconditionally; this will remove a lot of the stress in your life.

Spending time on yourself and learning to relax will also help your inner strength; many complementary therapies can help you here, such as aromatherapy, massage, yoga and reflexology.

Psychologically, this can help to support you. It's important to visualise yourself as a survivor rather than a victim of cancer; this will empower you to deal with the causes of your cancer and any side-effects that occur during your treatment.

And finally, having faith in some kind of supreme being or goodness – whether you like to call it God, an angel or by some other name – can also give you tremendous spiritual, psychological and emotional support when you're coming to terms with cancer.

Decreasing expenditure

With any form of credit, you have to pay back the principal plus interest. It's as true of nutritional energy (or 'money in to the energy bank') as it is of money. So the quickest way of decreasing your expenditure is to remove the need to pay back the extra interest – that is, removing the junk from your diet. This includes stimulants such as caffeine and alcohol, so-called energy products, refined and highly processed foods, and chemically isolated vitamins and minerals which your body simply can't use properly.

Looking at your lifestyle can help you see other ways of decreasing energy expenditure. If you habitually don't get enough sleep, eat *on the hoof*, rush around and don't give your body a chance to get a proper rest and do all the necessary repair work, you're depleting your energy reserves. Learn to manage your time so that you get whatever it is done without damaging your health.

Other energy depleters include smoking – acknowledged as one of the largest causes of cancer. If you don't smoke, your body doesn't have as many toxins to remove, and your energy levels will increase.

Net result

The net result of increasing your income and decreasing your expenditure is that all your direct debits dealing with digestion, assimilation, healing and repair will be met and your immune system and metabolism will function more effectively. And the level of your energy will rise consistently.

While cancer is a major problem when you have it – or have had it – don't forget that in the process of re-creating your health, any other problems which you may have had in the past and ignored will also benefit from the improvement in your health. The naturopathic approach is to treat the individual as a whole, not to concentrate on a specific disease: health is the removal of the causes of the disease, and once the causes of the disease have been removed, the symptoms will also disappear.

The right to choose

Above all, you have the right to choose the treatment that you feel is best for you. Don't allow anyone to rush you; and ask your practitioners as many questions as you need to make sure that you have all the information about the proposed treatment. Find out what all the options are: and, for each, what side-effects you're likely to encounter and how you can deal with them. If you want a second opinion, then ask for it. Only then will you be in a position to choose the treatment that is right for you.

The only real antidote to disease

Re-creation of health is exactly the same as preventing yourself getting cancer, either for the first time or for secondary cancer. The creation of health is the only real antidote to disease. So changing your lifestyle to improve the management of your nutrition, your bodily structure and your emotional/spiritual outlook will lead to a significantly more fulfilling future. There is an old Chinese saying that sums this up perfectly – and I leave you with this thought and my best wishes. 'Man is what he eats, what he drinks, how he breathes and how he thinks.'

Glossary of terms

Advanced Cancer
Where cancer that has spread from where it started to another part of the body.

Anaesthetic (general or local)
Drug which stops feeling, especially pain. General anaesthetics make you unconscious; local anaesthetics stop feeling in part of the body.

Anaemia
When your red blood cell count is low.

Angiogram
Also known as an arteriogram - where a special dye is injected into your artery and flows into the blood vessels, showing the position of the tumour when you are X-rayed.

Antibiotics
Drugs which fight bacterial infections.

Antibodies
Blood proteins produced by white blood cells when the body's immune system recognises an invader (e.g. bacteria). The antibodies attach themselves to the invader which is then destroyed.

Antiemetic
Anti-sickness drug.

Arteriogram
See angiogram

Axilla
Armpit.

B Lymphocytes (B cells)
Type of white blood cell that makes antibodies in response to disease or anything the body's immune system recognises as an invader.

Bacteria
Single cell micro-organisms which cause diseases if they get into the body.

Barium meal, barium enema
A white liquid used as a drink (barium meal) or passed by a tube into the back passage (barium enema). X-rays cannot go through it, so when the X-ray pictures are taken, the outline of the stomach or bowel shows up on the X-ray.

Benign
Not cancerous.

Bio-availability
Amount of the active ingredient of the vitamins or minerals that are absorbed by the body.

Biopsy
A piece of body tissue taken so that the cells can be looked at under a microscope.

Brachytherapy
See Internal Radiation.

Bronchoscope
A flexible tube with an eye piece and a light that enables doctors to see inside the windpipe (trachea) and the main airways of the lungs.

Bronchoscopy
A medical examination of the airways using a bronchoscope.

Carcinogen
Something that causes cancer.

Carcinoma
A cancer of the epithelial or skin tissue that covers all the body organs and lines all the body cavities. Most cancers are carcinomas.

Cell (Cells)
The building block of the body.

Chemosurgery
Repeated application of a chemical to the surface of a tumour to destroy it.

Chemotherapy
Drug treatment – usually used to mean with anti-cancer drugs.

Colon (Bowel, Large Bowel, Large Intestine)
Last part of the digestive system. Also called the large bowel, large intestine, or the bowel. Waste left from digested food passes through the bowel to the rectum (back passage) and then through the anus to the outside of the body.

Colonoscope
A long thin bendy tube connected to an eye-piece which allows the doctor to see inside the bowel.

Colonoscopy (Colonoscope)
Examination of the colon (large bowel) using a colonoscope.

Colostomy
Opening of the bowel onto the surface of the abdomen.

Craniotomy
A surgical opening in the scull when operating for brain cancer.

Cryosurgery
Freezing of a tomour using liquid nitrogen to destroy it.

CT Scan (CAT scan)
Computerised tomography scan; uses x-rays and a computer to construct pictures of the body in cross section.

Cystoscope
An instrument for looking at the inside of the bladder, the prostate gland and urethra.

Cystoscopy
Examination of the bladder and urethra using a cystoscope.

Cytotoxic
'Toxic to cells' – anti-cancer treatment.

Early Cancer
Cancer diagnosed at an early stage – i.e. a small tumour that has not spread.

Electrocautery
also known as electrosurgery. Use of a high-frequency current to kill cancer cells.

Endoscopy
Examination of your r colon through a special tube (an endoscope).

Enzyme (Enzymes)
Proteins that control chemical reactions in the body.

External Radiotherapy
Treatment with high energy waves which are beamed at a cancer (or the area where a cancer was) from outside the body.

Gene (Genes)
Coded messages made of DNA that tell cells how to behave and so control the growth and development of the body.

Grade
What the cancer cells look like under the microscope. The less they look like normal cells, the higher grade the cancer is said to be. Low grade cancers are likely to grow more slowly and be less likely to spread.

Haematoma
Swelling where blood has collected under the skin.

Hormone
Natural chemicals made in one part of the body which travel in the bloodstream and make things happen in another part of the body.

Interferon
Hormone-like substance produced by white blood cells to help your immune system fight infections; used to shrink tumours.

Internal Radiotherapy
Radiotherapy given by putting a source of radiation inside the body. Sometimes called 'brachytherapy'.

Intravenous Urogram
Scan of the kidneys, ureters, bladder and urethra.

Lobectomy
An operation to remove a lobe of an organ e.g. to remove a lobe of a lung.

Local Spread (Local Invasion)
Growth of a cancer into the area of the body around where it started.

Low Blood Count (Low Blood Counts)
Lower than normal levels of red or white blood cells, or platelets. Measured by a blood test.

Lumpectomy
Operation to remove a lump (usually breast).

Lymph
Body fluid which circulates through the lymphatic system. Carries food supplies to, and waste products away from, the body tissues.

Lymphangiogram (Lymphogram)
X-ray scan of the lymph glands using dye injected into the bloodstream.

Lymphatic System
System of tubes and glands in the body which filters body fluid and fights infection.

Lymph Nodes
Glands found throughout the body, particularly in the armpits, neck and groin; they fight infection and filter body fluid.

Lymphocytes
Type of white blood cell. There are two types of lymphocytes, B lymphocytes and T lymphocytes. They are part of the body's defence against disease, the immune response. B lymphocytes produce antibodies, helped by T lymphocytes

Lymphoedema
Swelling (usually of an arm or leg) due to blockage of the lymph vessels.

Lymphoma
Cancer of the lymphatic system.

Macrophages
White blood cells found in the lymph nodes which swallow up and kill foreign cells, including cancer cells.

Magnetic Resonance Imaging (MRI, MRI scan)
Scan using magnetism to build up a picture of the organs inside the body.

Malignant
Cancerous.

Mammogram
X-ray examination of the breast to look for early signs of cancer.

Mastectomy
Operation to remove the breast.

Metastasis
Where cancer spreads from one part of the body to another.

Monounsaturated Fat
Type of unsaturated fat in the diet found mainly in olive oil. Unsaturated fats are found in vegetables and vegetable oils.

Needle Aspiration
Type of biopsy. A needle is put into the area to be examined to draw off cells, which are looked at under the microscope to see if any are cancerous.

Needle Biopsy
Sample of tissue taken with a needle and looked at under a microscope.

Oedema
Swelling round the site of an operation.

Omega-3 Unsaturated Fatty Acid
Type of fat found in oily fish.

Oncologist
Doctor who specialises in treating cancer.

Orchidectomy
Operation to remove a testicle.

Placebo
Dummy treatment.

Platelet (Platelets)
Type of blood cell that helps the blood to clot.

Primary cancer (Primary Tumour)
Where the cancer started. The type of cell that has become cancerous will be the primary cancer – for example, if a biopsy from the liver or lung contains cancerous breast cells, then the primary cancer is breast cancer.

Radiotherapy (Radiotherapy Treatment, Radium Treatment)
Cancer treatment using high energy waves similar to X-rays.

Sarcoma
Muscle cancer

Saturated Fat
Type of fat found in meat and dairy products.

Scan
Looking at the inside of the body from the outside to see if there is anything wrong (eg CAT scan or ultrasound).

Secondary Cancer (Secondaries)
Cancer spread – also known as metastasis.

Seroma
Collection of fluid under a wound after an operation.

Side Effects
Unwanted effects of medical treatment.

Staging
Classifying a cancer by looking at the size of the tumour and whether it has spread. Used to decide the best course of treatment.

Tamoxifen (Nolvadex, Tamofen)
Hormone treatment for breast cancer. Stops breast cancer cells from picking up oestrogen. Oestrogen can encourage breast cancer to grow.

T Lymphocytes (T cells)
Type of white blood cell which help make antibodies as part of the immune response.

Tumour
Cancerous lump.
Ultrasound (Ultrasound scan)
Scan using sound waves to build up a picture of the inside of the body.

Unsaturated Fat
Type of fat found mainly in vegetables and vegetable oils.

Urethra
Tube which carries urine from the bladder to the outside of body.

White Blood Cells
Cells in the blood which fight infection and produce antibodies.

X-ray
Form of radiation used for taking pictures or for radiotherapy.

Appendix 1
Where to find alternative and complementary practitioners

1. IN THE UNITED KINGDOM

GENERAL
British Complementary Medicine Association
Kensington House
33 Imperial Square
Cheltenham
GL50 1QZ
Tel: 01242 519911
Website http://www.bcma.co.uk

Council for Complementary & Alternative
Medicine
Park House
206-208 Latimer Road
London W10 6RE
Tel: 020 8735 0632
Please send an SAE for information

ACUPUNCTURE
British Acupuncture Association
34 Alderney Street
London
SW1V 4EU
Tel: 020 7834 1012

British Acupuncture Council
Park House
206-208 Latimer Road
London W10 6RE
Tel 020 8964 0222
Website http://www.acupuncture.org.uk

British Medical Acupuncture Society
12 Marbury House
Higher Whitley
Warrington
Cheshire WA4 4QW
Tel: 01925 730727
Website http://www.medical-acupuncture.co.uk

ALEXANDER TECHNIQUE
STAT (Society of Teachers of Alexander
Technique)
129 Camden Mews
London NW1 9AH
Tel: 020 7284 3338
Website www.stat.org.uk

AROMATHERAPY
International Society of Professional
Aromatherapists
ISPA House
82 Ashby Road
Hinckley
Leicestershire LE10 ISN
Tel: 01455 637987

International Federation of Aromatherapists,
182 Chiswick High Road,
London
W4 1PP
Tel: 020 8742 2605
Website www.int-fed-aromatherapy.co.uk

Aromatherapy Organisations Council
3 Latymer Close
Braybrooke
Market Harborough
Leics
LE16 8LN

BACH FLOWER REMEDIES
The Dr Edward Bach Foundation
The Bach Centre
Mount Vernon
Bakers Lane
Sotwell
Wallingford
Oxfordshire OX10 0PZ
Tel: 01491 834678
Website: www.bachcentre.com

COLOUR
The International Association of Colour
46 Cottenham Road
Histon
Cambridge
CB4 4ES
Tel: 01223 563403

HEALING
National Federation of Spiritual Healers
Old Manor Farm Studio
Church Street
Sunbury-on-Thames
Middlesex
TW16 6RG
Tel: 01932 783164
Website www.nfsh.org.uk/

Confederation of Healing Organisations
113 High Street
Berkhamstead
Hertfordshire HP4 2DJ
Tel: 01442 870660

British Alliance of Healing Organisations
3 Sandy Lane
Gisleham
Lowestoft
Suffolk
NR33 8EQ
Tel: 01502 742224

HERBALISM
National Institute of Medical Herbalists
56 Longbrook Street
Exeter
Devon
EX4 6AH
Tel: 01392 426022
(Send an SAE for a list of local practitioners)
Website www.btinternet.com/~nimh

General Council and Register of Consultant
Herbalists
Grosvenor House
40 Sea Way
Middleton-on-Sea
West Sussex
PO22 7SA

HOMEOPATHY
British Homeopathic Association
27a Devonshire Street
London
W1N 1RJ
Tel: 020 7935 2163

Society of Homeopaths
2 Artizan Road
Northampton
NN1 4HU
Tel: 01604 621400

UK Homeopathy Medical Association
6 Livingstone Road
Gravesend
Kent
DA12 5DZ
Tel: 01474 560336

KINESIOLOGY
The Association of Systematic Kinesiology
(A.S.K.)
39 Browns Road
Surbiton
Surrey
KT5 85T
Tel: 020 8399 3215
Website: www.kinesiology.co.uk

MAGNETIC
The British Biomagnetic Association
The Williams Clinic
31 St Marychurch Road
Torquay
Devon
TQ1 3JF
Tel: 01803 293346

MASSAGE
British Massage Therapy Council
Greenbank House
65A Adelphi Street
Preston
PR1 7BH
Tel: 01772 881063
Website: www.bmtc.co.uk

Massage Therapy Institute of Great Britain
PO Box 2726
London
NW2 3NR
Tel: 0208 2081607

NATUROPATHY
General Council and Register of Naturopaths
Goswell House
2 Goswell Road
Street
Somerset
BA16 0JG
Tel: 01458 840072
Website: www.naturopathy.org.uk

REFLEXOLOGY
Association of Reflexologists
27 Old Gloucester Street
London WC1N 3XX
Tel: 01273 492385
Website: www.reflexology.org/aor

The British Reflexology Association
Monks Orchard
Whitborne
Worcs WR6 5RB
For a list of practitioners, send a cheque for £2

REIKI
Reiki Association
Cornbrook Bridge House
Clee Hill
Ludlow
Shropshire
SY8 3QQ
Tel: 01584 891197
Website: www.reikiassociation.org.uk

YOGA
British Wheel of Yoga
1 Hamilton Place
Boston Road
Sleaford
Lincolnshire NG34 7ES
Tel: 01529 306851
Website: members.aol.com/wheelyoga/

2. IN AUSTRALIA
GENERAL

For advice on various complementary therapies,
contact
Australian Complementary Health Association
Ross House
4th Floor, 247 Flinders Lane
Melbourne
Victoria 3000 Australia
Tel: (03) 9650 5327
Website: http://home.vicnet.net.au/~acha

ACUPUNCTURE
Australian Acupuncture and Chinese Medicine
Association Ltd
PO Box 5142
West End
Queensland 4101, Australia
Tel: (07) 3846 5866
National practitioner referral service Freecall
1800 025 334 (within Australia only)
Website: www.acupuncture.org.au

ALEXANDER TECHNIQUE
Australian Society of Teachers of the Alexander
Technique
PO Box 716 Darlinghurst
New South Wales 2010
Tel: 03 8339 571
Website: www.alexandertechnique.au

AROMATHERAPY
International Federation of Aromatherapists
PO Box 2210
Central Park
Victoria 3145 Australia
Tel: 0409 539 403
Website: www.ifa.org.au/

COLOUR THERAPY
See New Zealand

FLOWER REMEDIES
Flowerbase
PO Box 112
Upper Ferntree Gully
Victoria 3156 Australia
Website: http://www.ozelink.com/flowerbase/

HERBALISM
National Herbalists Association of Australia
33 Reserve Street
Annandale
New South Wales 2038
Tel (02) 9560 7077
Website: www.nhaa.org.au

HOMEOPATHY
Australian Homoepathic Association
PO Box 396
Drummoyne
New South Wales
Australia 2047
Tel: +61 2 9719 2793
Website: horizen.com.au

Australian Institute of Homeopathy
21 Bulah Close
Berdwra Heights
New South Wales
Australia 2082

MASSAGE
Massage Association of Australia
P.O Box 1187
Camberwell
Victoria 3124
Australia
Tel: (03) 98857631
Website: www.maa.org.au

Association of Massage Therapists Australia
PO Box 627
South Yarra
Victoria 3141
Australia
Tel: 03 9510 3930
NATUROPATHY
Australian Naturopathic Practitioners
Association
1st Floor
609 Camberwell Road
Camberwell 3124
Australia
Tel: 03-9889-0334; toll-free 1800 422 885
Website: www.vicnet.net.au/~anpa

REFLEXOLOGY
Reflexology Association of Australia
PO Box 366
Cammeray
New South Wales 2062
Australia
Tel: 02 9918 9241
Website: http://raa.inta.net.au

REIKI
Australian School of Reiki
PO Box 440
Ramsgate 2217
New South Wales
Australia
Tel: 02 9546 3135
Website: www.australianschoolofreiki.com

YOGA
Yoga Synergy
PO Box 9
Waverley 2024
Australia
Tel: (02) 9389 7399
Website: www.yogasynergy.com.au

3. IN CANADA

ACUPUNCTURE
Acupuncture Canada
107 Lietch Drive
Grimsby
Ontario L3M 2T9
Tel: 1-905-309-3245
Website: www.acupuncture.ca

ALEXANDER TECHNIQUE
CANSTAT (Society of Teachers of Alexander
Technique)
465 Wilson Avenue
Toronto
Ontario
M3H 1T9
Tel: 1-416-631-8127
Website: www.canstat.ca

AROMATHERAPY
Canadian Federation of Aromatherapists (CFA)
843479 Oxford Rd
84, R.R.3
Lakeside
Ontario
Canada
N0M 2G0
Tel: (519) 475-9038; toll-free 1-888-340-4445

FLOWER ESSENCES
Flower essence society
PO Box 459
Nevada City
CA 95959
Tel: 800-736-9222 (US & Canada)
Website: www.flowersociety.org/

HERBALISM
Canadian Herb Society
c/o Audrey Ostrom
VanDusen Botanical Gardens
5251 Oak St
Vancouver
BC V6M 4H1
Canada
Tel: 604-224-0457
Website: www.herbsociety.ca

The Canadian Association of Herbal
Practitioners
921 17th Avenue SW
Calgary
Alberta
T2T 0A4
Canada
Tel: (403) 270-0936

HOMEOPATHY
Canadian Foundation for Homeopathic
Research and Development
PO Box 8213
Station F
Edmonton
Alberta
T6H 4P1

Canadian Society of Homeopathy
87 Meadowlands Drive West
Nepean
Ontario K2G 2R9

KINESIOLOGY
Ontario Kinesiology Association
6519-B Mississagua Road
Mississauga
Ontario L5N 1A6
Tel: 905-567-7194
Website: www.oka.on.ca

British Columbia Association of Kinesiologists
2800-515 West Hastings St
Vancouver
British Columbia
V6B 5K3
Tel: 604.291.5097
Website: www.bcak.bc.ca/

MASSAGE
Canadian Massage Therapist Alliance/Alliance
Canadienne de Massotherapeutes
365 Bloor Street East
Suite 1807
Toronto
Ontario
Canada M4W 3L4
Tel: (416) 968-2149
Website: www.collinscan.com/~collins/
clientspgs/cmtai.html

NATUROPATHY
Canadian Naturopathic Association
1255 Sheppard Ave East (at Leslie)
North York
Ontario
M2K 1E2
Tel: 416-496-8633
Website: www.naturopathicassoc.ca/

REFLEXOLOGY
Reflexology Association of Canada
PO Box 110
451 Turnberry St
Brussels
Ontario N0G 1M0
Tel: 519-887-9991

Reflexology Association of British Columbia
214-3707
Hamber Place
North Vancouver
British Columbia
V7G 2J4
Tel: 1 604 435 8325

REIKI
Canadian Reiki Association
Box 40026
RPO Marlee
Toronto
Canada M6B 4K4
Tel: (416) 783-9904
Website: www.reiki.ca

YOGA
International Yoga Teachers Association
Ms Marion Mc Connell
1227 Kensington Street
Penticton
BC
V2A 4N3

4. IN NEW ZEALAND

GENERAL
New Zealand Natural Health Practitioners
Accreditation Board
PO Box 37-491
Auckland 1
New Zealand

ACUPUNCTURE
New Zealand School of Acupuncture & TCM
PO Box 11076
Wellington
New Zealand
Tel: 64 4 801 6400
Website: www.acupuncture.co.nz

The New Zealand Register of Acupuncturists Inc
P O Box 9950
Wellington 6001
New Zealand
Tel: 64 04 476 4866; Freephone 0800
Acupuncture (0800 228 786)

AROMATHERAPY
Aromatherapy New Zealand
PO Box 47 470
Ponsonby
Auckland
New Zealand
Tel: 64 9 378-6962
Website: www.aroma.co.nz

COLOUR THERAPY
Brooker Colour Therapy
35 Wordswoth Street
Cambridge
New Zealand
Tel: 64 7 827 3730
Website: www.colour-
therapy.co.nz/html/world_wide.html

HERBALISM
Herb Federation of New Zealand
PO Box 4055
Nelson South
New Zealand
Tel: 03-5469121

HOMEOPATHY
New Zealand Council of Homoeopaths
PO Box 51-195
Tawa
Wellington
New Zealand
Website: www.homeopathy.co.nz/

New Zealand Homoeopathic Society
PO Box 67-095
Mt. Eden
Auckland 1003
New Zealand
Website: www.homeopathic.co.nz/nzhs.htm

KINESIOLOGY
Touch for Health Association-New Zealand
Jim Wickenden
15 Selkirk Rd
Mt Albert
Auckland
New Zealand
Tel: +64-9.849 20 56

MASSAGE
NZ Association of Therapeutic Massage
Practitioners
PO Box 375
Hamilton
New Zealand

NATUROPATHY
New Zealand Society of Naturopaths
Website: www.naturopath.org.nz

REFLEXOLOGY
New Zealand Reflexology Association
PO Box 31084
Auckland 9
New Zealand
Tel: 64 9 486 1918

REIKI
Reiki New Zealand Inc.
PO Box 60-226
Titirangi
Auckland
New Zealand
Email: reiki@ihug.co.nz

YOGA
International Yoga Teachers Association
Ms Jenny Fellows
127 Seatoun Heights Rd
Wellington 3
New Zealand

5. IN SOUTH AFRICA

GENERAL
Confederation of Complementary Health
Associations of South Africa
PO Box 2471
Clareinch
7740
South Africa

ACUPUNCTURE
Institute of Chinese Medicine and Acupuncture
Dr Mogamat Jerome Fredericks DA DMA
(Representative IICMA Africa)
17 Urania Street
Observatory 2198
Johannesburg
Republic of South Africa
Tel: (27) 11-6488361
Website: www.acupuncture.co.za

ALEXANDER TECHNIQUE
SASTAT (South African Society for the
Alexander Technique)
P O Box 135
Simon's Town 7995
South Africa
Tel: +27 21 780 9412

AROMATHERAPY
Association of Aromatherapists Southern Africa
The AOASA
P O Box 23924
Claremont 7735
Cape Town
RSA
Tel: (021) 531-7314

HEALING
The Traditional Healers Organisation
PO Box 330
Steenberg 7947
Cape Town
RSA

HERBALISM
The Herbal Association of SA
PO Box 1831
Escourt
KwaZulu-Natal 3310
RSA
Tel:
(033) 263-1227

HOMEOPATHY
Homoeopathic Association of South Africa W.
Cape
Dr A Trevor
3 Golden Grove
Rondebosch, 7700
Tel: 021 686 2557

KINESIOLOGY
Touch for Health Association South Africa and
South African Association of Specialised
Kinesiologists
14 Osborne Road
Claremont Cape 7700 RSA
Tel: +27-21.61 80 21

MASSAGE
Massage Therapy Association
PO Box 53320
Kenilworth 7745
Tel: (021) 671-5313

NATUROPATHY
SA Naturopathy Association
Tel: 011 622-6967

REFLEXOLOGY
S.A. Reflexology Society
PO Box 1780
New Germany, 3620
Kwazulu
Natal
South Africa
Tel: 031 72-8531

YOGA
Institute of Yoga Teachers
Ms Joan van Alphen
501 Herschel Oaks
Herschel Road, Claremont 7700
Cape Town

Satyam Yoga Centre
18 Banbury Street
Bryanston
Gauteng
South Africa
Tel: +27 11 706 1709
Website: www.yoga.co.za/main.htm

6. IN THE UNITED STATES

ACUPUNCTURE
American Association of Oriental Medicine
433 Front St.
Catasauqua
PA 18032
Tel: (610) 266-1433
Toll Free: 888-500-7999
Website: www.aaom.org/

American Academy of Medical Acupuncture
5820 Wiltshire Boulevard #500
Los Angeles
California 90036
Tel: 213-937-5514
Website: www.medicalacupuncture.org

ALEXANDER TECHNIQUE
The American Society for the Alexander
Technique (AmSAT)
30 North Maple
PO Box 60008
Florence
MA 01062
Tel: Toll free within US: (800) 473 0620; else
(413) 584-2359
Website: www.alexandertech.org

AROMATHERAPY
American Aromatherapy Association
P.O. Box 3679
South Pasadena
CA 91031
Tel: 818-457-1742

National Association for Holistic Aromatherapy
P.O. Box 17622
Boulder
CO 80308-0622
Tel: 303-258-3791

BACH FLOWER
American Council on Science and Health
1995 Broadway, 2nd Floor
New York
NY 10023
Tel: 212-362-7044
Website: www.acsh.org

Flower Essence Society
PO Box 459
Nevada City
CA 95959
Tel: 800-736-9222 (US & Canada)
Website: www.flowersociety.org

HEALING
American Association of Alternative Healers
PO Box 10026
Sedona
Arizona 86336-8026
Tel: 530-345-8622

HERBALISM
American Herbalists' Guild
1931 Gaddis Road
Canton
GA 30115
Tel: (770) 751-6021
Website: www.healthy.net/herbalists/

HOMEOPATHY
American Institute of Homeopathy
801 North Fairfax Street Suite 306
Alexandria
VA 22314
Tel: 703 246-9501
Website: www.homeopathyusa.org/

The National Center for Homeopathy
801 North Fairfax St. Suite 306
Alexandria
VA 22314
Tel: 703-548-7790
Website: www.homeopathic.org

KINESIOLOGY
American Kinesiotherapy Association
One IBM Plaza Suite 2500
Chicago
IL 60611
Tel: 800/296-AKTA
Website: www.akta.org

Association of Specialized Kinesiologists, ASK-US
Linda Clarke Scott (President)
4201 Wilson Blvd #110-395
Arlington
VA 22203-1859
Tel: +1-888-749-6464
Website: www.assn-ask-us.com

MAGNETIC
International Foundation of BioMagnetics
5447 East 5th Street
Suite 111
Tucson
Arizona 98816
Tel: 520-323-7951

MASSAGE
American Massage Therapy Association
820 Davis Street, Suite 100
Evanston
IL 60201-4444
Tel: 847/864-0123

International Massage Association
92 Main Street
PO Drawer 421
Warrenton
Virginia 20188
Tel: 540-351-0800

National Association of Massage Therapy
PO Box 1400
Westminster
Colorado 80030-1400
Tel: 800-776-6268

NATUROPATHY
The American Association of Naturopathic
Physicians
8201 Greensboro Drive
Suite 300
McLean
Virginia 22102
Tel: 703-610-9037
Website: www.naturopathic.org

American Naturopathic Medical Association
PO Box 96273
Las Vegas
Nevada 89193
Tel: (702) 897-7053
Website: www.anma.com

REFLEXOLOGY
American Reflexology Certification Board
(ARCB)
PO Box 620607
Littleton
CO 80162
Tel: 303-933-6921
Website: www.arcb.net

Reflexology Association of America
4012 S Rainbow Boulevard
K-PMB# K585
Las Vegas
Nevada 89103-2059
USA
Tel: 702-871-9522
Website: www.reflexology-usa.org

REIKI
The Reiki FoundationTM
PO Box 362
Brewster
NY 10509-0362
Tel (914)-278-3038
Websites: www.asunam.com/ or
www.asunam.com/reiki_foundation.htm

YOGA
American Yoga Association
PO Box 19986
Sarasota
FL 34276
Tel: (941) 927-4977
Website: www.americanyogaassociation.org

Appendix 2
RDA of vitamins and minerals for healthy adults and for adults with cancer

Vitamin/Mineral	Function in the body	RDA for healthy adult	Supplement recommended for adults with cancer
Vitamin A betacarotene, changed to retinal in the body)	Helps eyesight and skin; acts as antioxidant to neutralise free radicals	800 micrograms	366 micrograms
Vitamin B1 (Thiamin)	Makes energy available in the body and maintains a healthy nervous system	1.4 milligrams	0.7 milligrams
Vitamin B2 (Riboflavin)	Forms flavin adenine dinucleotide and flavin mononuclotide to help make energy available in the body	1.6 milligrams	0.8 milligrams
Vitamin B6	Acts with enzymes to regulate chemical reactions in the body; needed to form haemoglobin, antiobodies and neurotransmitters	2 milligrams	20–30 milligrams
Vitamin B12	Recycles enzymes; makes red blood cells; insulates nerve cells	1 microgram	0.5 micrograms
Vitamin C	Antioxidant; helps form collagen (in the skin) and helps the body absorb iron	60 milligrams	30 milligrams
Vitamin D	Helps the body absorb and use calcium	5 micrograms	2.5 micrograms

Vitamin/Mineral	Function in the body	RDA for healthy adult	Supplement recommended for adults with cancer
Vitamin E	Antioxidant; protects cell membranes, maintains healthy skin	10 milligrams	3.3 milligrams
Vitamin K	Regulates blood clotting and helps maintenance of bones and teeth	None	0.02 milligrams
Biotin	Regulates enzymes – particularly those in the release of energy from food	0.15 milligrams	0.075 milligrams
Boron	Helps the body use calcium	None	0.5 milligrams
Calcium	Needed to build and maintain bones and teeth	800 milligrams	9 milligrams
Choline	Maintains proper functioning of gall bladder and liver, breaks down fats in liver and assists transmission of nerve pulses.	–	2.5 milligrams
Chromium	Involved in the processes that make glucose available for energy and in the metabolism of amino acids and fats	None	25 micrograms
Copper	Proteins involved in growth, nerve function and energy release	None	0.25 milligrams
Folic acid	Formation of red blood cells	200 micrograms	100 micrograms
Inositol	Combines with fatty acids to form phospholipids, needed to form cell membranes	None	2.5 milligrams
Iodine	Used to form thyroid hormones which regulate the body's metabolic rate	150 micrograms	75 micrograms
Iron	Used to form haemoglobin	14 milligrams	7.50 milligrams
Magnesium	Used for enzyme regulation, healthy nerves and muscles, helps calcium move into the bones	300 milligrams	3 milligrams
Manganese	Needed to form enzymes	None	0.25 milligrams

Vitamin/Mineral	Function in the body	RDA for healthy adult	Supplement recommended for adults with cancer
Molybdenum	Needed to form enzymes, particularly for breaking down waste products in urine	None	15 micrograms
Niacin	Helps release energy from food	18 milligrams	9 milligrams
Pantothenic acid	Helps release energy from food	6 milligrams	3 milligrams
Para-aminobenzoic acid	Keeps hair colour in tact, protects from harmful rays of the sun and aids formation of red blood cells.	–	2.5 milligrams
Phosphorus	Makes calcium stable to build and maintain bones and teeth; helps release energy from food	800 milligrams	3 milligrams
Potassium	Helps maintain cell health and transmission of signals in nerves and muscles	None	3 milligrams
Selenium	Forms enzymes and acts as an antioxidant	None	149 micrograms
Zinc	Tissue growth, maintenance of the immune system and maintenance of healthy skin, hair and nails	15 milligrams	2.5 milligrams

Appendix 3
Approximate correlation between food state nutrients and traditional supplements

There is no direct unvarying, equivalent ration between food state vitamins and minerals and traditional supplements, particularly as the individual's level of bio-availability differs from day to day.
In my experience, however, the approximate relation between the two are as follows:

Vitamin/mineral	Food state	Traditional supplement
Betacarotene (Vitamin A)	4.5 mg	6 mg (10,000-12,000 iu)
Thiamin (Vitamin B1)	25 mg	50-60 mg
Riboflavin (Vitamin B2)	20 mg	40-50 mg
Niacin (Vitamin B3)	50 mg	100-150 mg
Pantothenic Acid (Vitamin B5)	50 mg	100-120 mg
Vitamin B6	20 mg	40-50 mg
Vitamin C	250 mg	750-1000 mg
Vitamin E	150 iu	800-1000 iu
Calcium	30 mg	200-300 mg: varies depending on material used, but roughly equivalent to 100 mg elemental of an inorganic salt of calcium
Iron/Molybdenum	5mg/10mcg	10-12mg (elemental iron; does not apply to simple ferrous salts such as ferrous sulphate)
Chromium	60 mcg	No similar material available for comparison
Magnesium	30mg	Around 100mg
Potassium	30 mg	Around 150-200 mg
Selenium	100mcg	No comparable form
Zinc/copper	15mg/1mg	Around 100mg (orotate)

Appendix 4
Cancer help groups

IN THE UK

GENERAL
Bristol Cancer Help Centre
Grove House,
Cornwallis Grove, Clifton,
Bristol BS8 4PG
Tel: 0117 980 9500
Website: www.bristolcancerhelp.org

CancerBACUP - British Association of Cancer
United Patients
Cancer Information Service
3 Bath Place, London EC2A 3JR
Counselling service: 020 7696 9000
Cancer information service (staffed by special-
ist cancer nurses): 020 7613 2121 or freephone
0800 181199
Website http://www.cancerbacup.org.uk

Macmillan Cancer Relief
Helpline: 0845 601 6161, Mondays to Fridays,
9.30-7.30 pm
Website: www.macmillan.org.uk

BLADDER CANCER
The Continence Foundation
307 Hatton Square, 16 Baldwins Gardens,
London EC1N 7RJ
Helpline: 020 7 831 9831 (9.30am - 4.30pm
Monday to Friday)
Website: www.vois.org.uk/cf/

Urostomy Association
Central Office
'Buckland'
Beaumont Park
Danbury
Essex
CM3 4DE
Tel: 0124 541 4294
Website www.uagbi.org

BOWEL CANCER
Beating Bowel Cancer (formerly the Crocus
Trust)
PO Box 360
Twickenham
TW1 1UN
Tel: 020 8892 5256
Website: www.beatingbowelcancer.org

British Colostomy Association
15 Station Road
Reading
Berkshire
RG1 1LG
Tel: 0118 939 1537 or freephone helpline: 0800
3284257
Website www.bcass.org.uk

Colon Cancer Concern
4 Rickett Street
London
SW6 1RU
Infoline: 020 7381 4711 Mon-Fri 10am-4pm
24hr answerphone.
Website: www.coloncancer.org.uk

BRAIN CANCER
Brain Tumour Action
Norton Park
57 Albion Road
Edinburgh
EH7 5QY
Tel: 0131 466 0236
Website: www.cancerpoint.org/bta/

United Kingdom Brain Tumour Society
BAC House
Bonehurst Road
Horley
Surrey RH6 8QG
Tel: 01252 653807

BREAST CANCER
Breast Cancer Campaign
Breast Cancer Campaign
Stapleton House
29-33 Scrutton Street
London EC2A 4HU
Tel: 020 7749 3700
Website: www.bcc-uk.org

Breast Cancer Care
Kiln House
210 New Kings Road
London
SW6 4NZ
Helpline: 0808 800 6000
Website: www.breastcancercare.org.uk

National Hereditary Breast Cancer Helpline
Tel: 01629 813000

CERVICAL CANCER
GYNAE C
1 Bolingbroke Road
Swindon
Wiltshire SN2 2LB
Tel: 01793 338885

LUNG CANCER
British Lung Foundation
78 Hatton Garden
London
EC1N 8LD
Tel: 020 7831 5831
Website: www.lunguk.org/index.htm

Roy Castle Lung Cancer Foundation
200 London Road
Liverpool L3 9TA
Helpline: 0800 358 7200
Website: www.roycastle.org

LYMPHOMA CANCER
Leukaemia Research Fund
43 Great Ormond Street
London WC1N 3JJ
Tel: 020 7405 0101
Website: www.leukaemia-research.org.uk

Lymphoma Association
PO Box 386
Haddenham
Aylesbury
HP20 2GA
Tel: 0808 808 5555
Website: www.lymphoma.org.uk

PROSTATE CANCER
Men's Health Matters
Blythe Hall
100 Blythe Road
London
W14 0HB
Tel: 020 8995 4448 (lines manned between
6.00pm - 8.00pm weekdays)
Website: www.macmillan.org.uk/framea.html

Prostate Cancer Charity
Du Cane Road
London
W12 ONN
Helpline: 0208 383 1948
Website: www.prostate-cancer.org.uk

SKIN CANCER
MARCS (Melanoma and Related Cancers of the
Skin)
Marc's Line Resource Centre
Dermatology Treatment Centre
Level 3
Salisbury District Hospital
Salisbury
SP2 8BJ
Tel: 01722 415071
Website: www.k-web.co.uk

TESTICULAR CANCER
The Orchid Cancer Appeal
Dept of Medical Oncology
St Bartholomew's Hospital
1st Floor King George V Building
West Smithfield
London
EC1A 7BE
Tel: 020 7601 8522
Website: www.orchid-cancer.org.uk

AMERICA

GENERAL
American cancer society
Website: www.cancer.org
Tel: call 1-800-ACS-2345 (offices in every state)

National Cancer Institute
Tel: 1-800-4-CANCER (1–800–422–6237)
Monday–Friday 9am–4.30 pm
Website: www.nci.nih.gov

BLADDER CANCER
American Foundation for Urologic Disease
1128 North Charles Street
Baltimore
Maryland 21201
Tel: 410-468-1800
Website: www.afud.org

BOWEL CANCER
Colon Cancer Alliance
175 Ninth Avenue
New York
NY 10011
Toll-free helpline: 1-877-422-2030
Website: www.ccalliance.org

BRAIN CANCER
American Brain Tumor Assocation
2720 River Road
Des Plaines
IL 60018
Tel: (847) 827-9910
Patient Line: (800) 886-2282
Website: www.abta.org

BREAST CANCER
National Alliance of Breast Cancer Organisation
9 East 37th Street
New York
NY 10016
Tel: (212) 889-0606
Website: www.nabco.org

CERVICAL CANCER
National Cervical Cancer Coalition (NCCC)
16501 Sherman Way
Suite # 110
Van Nuys, Ca† 91406
Tel: (800) 685-5531
Website: www.nccc-online.org

LUNG CANCER
Alliance for lung cancer
PO Box 849
Vancouver
WA 98666
USA
Tel: (800) 298-2436 (US only) or (360) 696-2436.
Website: www.alcase.org

LYMPHOMA CANCER
Lymphoma Research Foundation of America
8800 Venice Boulevard
Suite 207
Los Angeles
CA 90034
Tel: (310) 204-7040
Website: www.lymphoma.org

PROSTATE CANCER
National Prostate Cancer Coalition
1156 15th Street
Suite 905
Washington
DC 20005
Tel: (202) 463 9455

Prostate Cancer Support Network
1218 North Charles Street
Baltimore
MD 21201
Tel: (800) 828 7866

SKIN CANCER
Melanoma Research Foundation
23704-5 El Toro Rd., #206
Lake Forest
CA 92630
Tel: 1-800-MRF-1290
Website: www.melanoma.org

AUSTRALIA

GENERAL
Australian Cancer Society
PO Box 4708
Sydney
NSW 2001
Tel: + 61 2 9380 9022
Website: www.cancer.org.au

Anti-Cancer Foundation of SA
202 Greenhill Road
PO Box 929
Eastwood SA 5063
Unley SA 5061
Tel: [08] 8291 4111; cancer helpline [08] 8291
4111 local callers, [1800] 188 070 country
callers

BREAST CANCER
National Breast Cancer Centre
PO Box 572
Kings Cross
NSW 1340
Australia
Tel: (02) 9334 1700,
Website: www.nbcc.org.au

LYMPHOMA CANCER
Lymphoedema Association of Australia
94 Cambridge Terrace
Malvern
SA 5061
Tel: 61+(8) 8271-2198
Website: www.lymphoedema.org.au

PROSTATE CANCER
Prostate Cancer Foundation Of Australia
PO Box 1332
Lane Cove
NSW, 1595
Hotline: 1-800-22-00-99 (Australia only)

Tel: +61-2-9418-7942
Website: www.prostate.org.au/

SKIN CANCER
SunSmart – Anti-Cancer Council of Victoria
1 Rathdowne Street
Carlton, Victoria
Australia 3053
Tel: 61 (03) 9635 5148
Website: www.sunsmart.com.au

Skin cancer Research Foundation (SA)
Tel: 61 8 8239 1531
Email: uvray@gist.net.au
Website: skincancer.cool.net.au

NEW ZEALAND

GENERAL
Cancer Society of New Zealand
PO Box 12145
Wellington
Toll-free information service tel: 0800 800 426
Website: www.cancernz.org.nz/

BREAST CANCER
Breast Health New Zealand
Website: www.breast.co.nz/

CANADA

GENERAL
National Cancer Institute of Canada
Suite 200
10 Alcorn Avenue
Toronto Ontario
M4V 3B1
Tel: 416-961-7223; Cancer Information Service
tollfree 1-888-939-3333 (Monday to Friday,
9am–6pm, bilingual).
Website: www.ncic.cancer.ca

BOWEL CANCER
Colorectal Cancer Association of Canada
Ottawa Regional Cancer Center
501 Smyth Road
Ottawa
Ontario K1H 8L6
Tel: toll-free 1-888-318-9442
Website: www.ccac-accc.ca

BREAST CANCER
Breast Cancer Society of Canada
401 St. Clair Street
Point Edward
Ontario N7V 1P2
National Toll Free: 1.800.567.8767
Website: HYPERLINK http://www.bcsc.ca/
 www.bcsc.ca/

Canadian Breast Cancer Foundation
790 Bay Street
Suite 1000
Toronto
ON M5G 1N8
Tel: (416) 596-6773 or toll-free 1 (800) 387-
9816
Website: www.cbcf.org

LYMPHOMA CANCER
Lymphoma Foundation Canada
63 Havelock St
Toronto
Ontario
M6H 3B3
Website: http://www.canlymphomafounda-
tion.org

PROSTATE CANCER
The National Association of Prostate Cancer
Support Groups
PO Box 1253
Lakefield
ON
K0L 2H0

SOUTH AFRICA

GENERAL
Cancer Association of South Africa
Tel: 0800 226622 (toll-free)
Website: www.cansa.org.za

Appendix 5
Suppliers

1. FOOD STATE NUTRIENTS

UK
Nature's Own
Unit 8
Hanley Workshops
Hanley Road
Hanley Swan
Worcestershire
WR8 0DX
Tel: 01684 310022

SOUTH AFRICA
Sportron International
6 Cambridge Park
22 Witkoppen Road
Paulshof
Sandton
South Africa
Tel: 002711 259 2200

Food State Nutrients
P.T.Y. Limited
c/o Sportron International
6 Cambridge Park
22 Witkoppen Road
Paulshof
Sandton
South Africa
0027118072728

USA
Sportron U.S.A.
115 Industrial Boulevard
Suite B, McKinney
Texas 75069
Tel: 001 972 509 1234

AUSTRALIA AND NEW ZEALAND
As UK

CANADA
Harlon Lati
Sisu Enterprises Co Ltd
104a - 3430 Brighton Street
Burnaby
BCV5A3H4
Canada
Tel: 0016044206610

2. RAPHA

Rapha UK
1 The Stables
Walwyn Road
Colwall
Worcs
WR13 6QZ
El 01684 541262
Website www.rapha.com

Index

Acupuncture 78–9
Alexander technique 79–80, 174
Alkylating agents 55
Alternative therapies
  approach of 89
  colonic irrigation 76
  diet, restriction of 76
  Gerson system 76
  hydrotherapeutic techniques 76
  practitioners 195–204
  purpose of 75
Angels 180–1
Angiogram 36
Antibiotics
  animal development, use in 99
  chemotherapy, use for 56
  overuse of 22
Antimetabolites 56
Aromatherapy 80
Arteriogram 36
Avocado
  bean and avocado salad 128
  cold tomato and avocado soup 120
  guacamole 146

Bach flower remedies 81
Barium enema 34
Bean and avocado salad 128
Biomagnetic energy 23
Biopsies 36
Bladder cancer
  chemotherapy 59, 69
  diagnosis 44
  facts and figures 38
  radiotherapy 59, 69
  side-effects 69
  surgery 58, 68
  warning signs 41
Bowel cancer
  chemotherapy 60, 69
  diagnosis 44
  facts and figures 38
  radiotherapy 60, 69
  side-effects 69
  surgery 60, 69
  warning signs 41
Brain cancer
  chemotherapy 61, 70
  diagnosis 45
  facts and figures 38
  radiotherapy 61, 70
  side-effects 70–1
  surgery 61, 70
  warning signs 41–2
Breast cancer
  chemotherapy 63, 71
  diagnosis 45
  facts and figures 39
  hormone drugs, use of 63, 71
  lumpectomy 62
  mastectomy 62
  radiotherapy 62, 71
  self-examination 34
  side-effects 70–1
  surgery 62, 70
  warning signs 42
Breathing exercises 163–4
Bristol Cancer Help Centre 177
Broccoli and tofu stir-fry with peanut sauce
  140

Cabbage
  robust cabbage and raisin salad 129
Cancer see also Breast cancer, etc
  biopsies 36
  cells, development of 32
  civilisation, as disease of 20
  control over 19
  crisis, as 14
  detecting 33
  emotional, physical and spiritual lessons

165–76
epidemic proportions, reaching 20
full information service, need for 92
management, decisions for 15
people with 178
scans 34–6
screening 34
self-examination 34
signs of 33
treatment see Treatment
Cancer Help Centre 177
Cancer help groups 209–13
Caponata 124
Castle, Roy 27
Cauliflower and mushrooms in black bean
   sauce 139
Cervical cancer
   chemotherapy 64, 72
   diagnosis 45
   facts and figures 39
   radiotherapy 63, 71
   side-effects 72
   surgery 63, 71
   warning signs 42
Chemical energy 23
Chemosurgery 50
Chemotherapy
   cancers responding to 55
   combination drugs 55
   drugs, use of 54–5
   forms of drugs 56
   immune system, damage to 90
   matters taken into account 55
   purpose of 30
   side-effects 56–8
      avoiding 90
   specific use of see Bladder cancer, etc
Chemotherapy diet 105
Chestnut and Brussels Sprout soup 121
Chinese medical system 20
Cold vaporisation 114–115
Colonic irrigation 76
Colostomy 51
Colour therapy 81–2
Complementary therapies
   acupuncture 78–9
   Alexander technique 79–80
   approach of 89

aromatherapy 80
Bach flower remedies 81
benefits of 92
colour therapy 81–2
destressing, for 175
healing 82–3
health, re-creation of 91, 93
herbalism 83
homeopathy 84–5
kinesiology 85
magnetic therapy 86
massage 86
practitioners 195–204
purpose of 75
reflexology 87
reiki 88
side-effects, avoiding 90
yoga 88–9
Counselling 173
Crisis
   definition 14, 19
   different way of life, leading to 177
Cryosurgery 50
CT scan 35

Dairy produce 102
Dehydration 112–13
Destressing techniques
   Alexander technique 174
   complementary therapies 175
   Eeman technique 173
Detoxification 107
Diagnosis 17
   bladder cancer 44
   bowel cancer 44
   brain cancer 45
   breast cancer 45
   cervical cancer 45
   coping with 47
   lung cancer 46
   lymphoma cancer 46
   prostate cancer 46
   skin cancer 46
   testicular cancer 46
Disease
   reversal of process 31
   treatment 30

Eeman technique 173
Electrocautery 50
Electrosurgery 50
Energy
  bank 27–30, 186
  biomagnetic 23
  body function, as key to 22
  borrowing 28
  chemical 23
  elimination 101
  emotional 188
  equation 24–5
  expenditure, decreasing 188–9
  imbalance 26
  income, increasing 187–8
  levels, drop in 22
  life 24–5
  loss of, effect 29
  nutritional 187
  obstructions 24–6
  ongoing activities 28
  psychological, emotional and spiritual
    obstructions 188
  rebuilding 30
  resonant 23
  source of 22
  structural 187
Exercise
  abdominal press 157
  alternate knee raises 160
  arm stretch 158
  arm swinging 159
  breathing exercises 163–4
  cancer, while suffering from 154–5
  cat stretch 157
  chest raises 162–3
  fit, when 160–3
  forehead to knee 159
  hip circling 156
  hip stretch 160
  increasing 158–60
  kneeling press-ups 157
  leg lifts 162–3
  neck stretch 156
  need for 153
  nutrition and emotional state, interaction
    with 153
  opposite arm and leg stretch 159

  sensible 154
  sex 164
  shrugging 157
  side stretching 156
  sit-ups to alternate knee 162
  sit-ups to both knees 162
  starting 155–8
  trunk twisting 158
  walking 154

Fear 165–68
Fertilisers
  artificial and organic 100
Food see Nutrition
Fos-a-dophilus 115
Future, looking to 165

Gerson system 76
Glossary 191–94
Guacamole 146

Healing
  ancient and current wisdom 15
  naturopathic approach 15, 16
  process of 82
  therapy, as 82–3
Health
  normal 19
  personal responsibility for 31
  re-creation of 91, 93, 103–7, 186
  symptom removal, focus on 21
Herbalism 83
Hippocrates 94
Homeopathy 84–5
Hormones
  breast cancer, treatment of 63, 71
  chemotherapy, use for 56
  prostate cancer, treatment of 67, 74
Hydrotherapeutic techniques 76

Immune system
  cancer cells, controlling 21–22
  chemotherapy, damage by 90
  function, lowering 21–22

Jerusalem artichoke soup 120

Kinesiology 85

Lasagne 130
Laser surgery 50
Leeks, braised 145
Lentils
  braised lentils and bulgur wheat 135
  lentil bake with almond sauce 136
  lentil, tomato and barley soup 118
Life energy 24–5
Life, understanding of 182
Listening, importance of 180
Liver
  wastes, elimination 101
Love
  present of 170–2
  relationships of 170–2
  responsibility for 170–2
Lumpectomy 62
Lung cancer
  chemotherapy 65, 73
  diagnosis 46
  facts and figures 39
  non-small lung cell 64–5
  radiotherapy 65, 73
  side-effects 73
  small lung cell 65
  surgery 64–5, 73
  warning signs 42
Lymphangiogram 36
Lymphoma cancer
  chemotherapy 66, 73
  diagnosis 46
  facts and figures 40
  interferon, use of 66, 73
  radiotherapy 65, 73
  side-effects 73
  warning signs 43
  watchful waiting 65

Magnetic therapy 86
Massage 86
Mastectomy 62
Medicine
  history, in 20
  today 21
Metastasis 37
Middle Eastern bread salad 127
Middle Eastern tomato salad 125
Minerals

absorption and bio-availability 94–7
food state 109, 208
functions 210–12
meat, poultry and fish, in 97
recommended daily allowances 205–7
replacing in soil 95–6
soil structure, changing 95–6
supplements 109, 215
vegetables, in 96
water, in 98
Misdiagnosis 17
MRI scan 35
Mushrooms
  braised lentils, mushrooms and shallots with
    bulgur wheat 135
  cauliflower and mushrooms in black bean
    sauce 141
  Chinese egg noodles with mushrooms 133

Naturopathy
  healing, approach to 15, 16
  mental approach, changing 18
  orthodox approach distinguished 16–17
  principles 16
Naturotherapy
  alternative approach, offering 76
  case histories 77–8
  diet, restriction of 76–7
  individual, responsibility of 78
  problem with 78
  side-effects, avoiding 90
Negativity 170
Nutrition
  animal foods 98–99
  artificial and organic fertilisers 99
  baking 109
  balance of foodstuffs 101–3
  blackened foods 109
  body, use by 111
  boiling 109
  chemical energy, as 23
  chemotherapy diet 105
  dairy produce 102
  detoxification 107
  eating for health 117
  eating in season 100
  eating to get well 115–117
  exercise and emotional state, interaction with

155
food preparation 107–9
general diet 105-7
grilling 108
health, re-creation of 103–7
healthy approach 109
junk, removing 187
microwaving 109–10
minerals 94–7 see also Minerals
organic foods 100
proteins 102
quality food, obtaining 94
raw foods 108
recipes see Recipes
steaming 108
stir-frying 108
supplementation 109–11, 115–17, 208
wastes, elimination 101
water see Water

Oncologist, seeing 48
Organic foods 77, 100
Osmosis, reverse 114
Oxidisation 100–1

Pasta
  Chinese egg noodles with mushrooms 133
  lasagne 130
  pasta Siciliana 132
  roasted tomato and pasta salad 124
Plant alkaloids 56
Positive thinking
  mind, using 170
  optimism 170
  people around, by 171–3
  within oneself 170
Posture 151–2, 187
Potage Bonne Femme 119
Present, living in 168
Pro-biotics 115
Prostate cancer
  chemotherapy 67
  diagnosis 46
  facts and figures 40
  hormone therapy 67, 74
  radiotherapy 66–7, 74
  side-effects 74
  surgery 66, 73

warning signs 43
watchful waiting 66
Proteins 102

Radiotherapy
  brachytherapy 52
  external beam radiation 51
  good cells, destroying 52
  internal beam radiation 52
  purpose of 30
  scarring 54
  side-effects 53–4
  side-effects, avoiding 90
  specific use of see Bladder cancer, etc
  types of 51–52
  use of 52
Recipes
  baked peaches 148
  baked rice and peas 123
  bean and avocado salad 128
  braised leeks 145
  braised lentils with bulgur wheat 135
  broccoli and tofu stir-fry with peanut sauce
    140
  caponata 122
  cauliflower and mushrooms in black bean
    sauce 139
  chestnut and Brussels Sprout soup 121
  Chinese egg noodles with mushrooms 133
  cold tomato and avocado soup 120
  guacamole 146
  Jerusalem artichoke soup 120
  lasagne 130
  lentil bake with almond sauce 136
  lentil, tomato and barley soup 118
  Middle Eastern bread salad 127
  Middle Eastern tomato salad 125
  pasta Siciliana 132
  perfumed tofu 134
  plum crumble 150
  potage Bonne Femme 119
  raisin and hazelnut pudding 149
  red bean dip 147
  roasted tomato and pasta salad 124
  roasted vegetables with smoked tofu 138
  robust cabbage and raisin salad 131
  saffron lentils 144
  spicy potato curry 143

tasty rice salad 126
tricolour pepper salad 124
wilted greens 146
winter roasted squash with peanut sauce 142
Red bean dip 147
Reflection, traditions of 182
Reflexology 87
Reiki 88
Religion 175–76
Resonant energy 23
Rice
baked rice and peas 123
tasty rice salad 126
Roasted tomato and pasta salad 124
Rollason, Helen 77

Salads
bean and avocado salad 128
Middle Eastern bread salad 127
roasted tomato and pasta salad 124
robust cabbage and raisin salad 131
tasty rice salad 126
tricolour pepper salad 124
Scans
angiogram 36
arteriogram 36
barium enema 34
CT scan 35
lymphangiogram 36
MRI 35
ultrasound 36
X-rays 35
Screening 33–4
Self-examination 34
Sex 164
Skin cancer
chemotherapy 68
diagnosis 46
facts and figures 40–1
side-effects 74
surgery 67, 74
warning signs 43
Smoking 26–7, 189
Soil structure, changing 95–7
Soup
chestnut and Brussels Sprout soup 121
cold tomato and avocado soup 120
Jerusalem artichoke soup 120

lentil, tomato and barley soup 118
potage Bonne Femme 119
Spicy potato curry 143
Spine 156
Staging 37–8
Stress 26
removing 173 see also Destressing techniques
Structure 152
Supplementation 109–11, 115–17, 208
Surgery
chemosurgery 50
colostomy 51
cryosurgery 50
electrocautery 50
electrosurgery 50
laser 50
postural problems 51
psychological problems 51
purpose of 30
reconstructive 50
side-effects 51
specific use of see Bladder cancer, etc

Testicular cancer
chemotherapy 68
diagnosis 46
facts and figures 41
self-examination 34
side-effects 74
surgery 68, 74
warning signs 43
Tofu
broccoli and tofu stir-fry with peanut sauce 140
perfumed tofu 134
roasted vegetables with smoked tofu 138
Tomatoes
cold tomato and avocado soup 120
lentil, tomato and barley soup 118
roasted tomato and pasta salad 124
Treatment
approach of 89
cause removal techniques 89
chemotherapy 54–8 see also Chemotherapy
choice, making 48, 189–90
decisions, time for 47
improvements in 58
orthodox 17, 49
radiotherapy 51–3 see also Radiotherapy

side-effects 68–74
surgery 49–51 see also Surgery
Tricolour pepper salad 126

Ultrasound scan 36

Vegans 103
Vegetables
  caponata 124
  roasted vegetables with smoked tofu 140
Vegetarians 103
Vinca alkaloids 56
Vitamins
  food state 111, 208
  functions 205–07
  need for 103, 189
  recommended daily allowances 205–07
  supplements 109

Walking 154
Wallace, Peter 177
Wastes, elimination 101
Water
  bottled 112–13
  cold vaporisation 114–15
  distilled 113–14
  filtered 113
  importance of 112
  plant cycle, in 98
  reverse osmosis 114
  tap 112
Wilted greens 147
Winter roasted squash with peanut sauce 144

X–rays 35

Yoga 88–9